EVERYDAY PEDIATRICS

Everyday Pediatrics

🦎 ELMER R. GROSSMAN, M.D.

W.B. Saunders Company
A Division of Harcourt Brace & Company

Philadelphia   London   Toronto
Montreal   Sydney   Tokyo

W.B. Saunders Company
A Division of Harcourt Brace & Company

The Curtis Center
Independence Square West
Philadelphia, PA 19106

Photograph by Jo Brocone and Nick Smee. Tony Stone Images.

Library of Congress Cataloging-in-Publication Data

Grossman, Elmer R.
    Everyday pediatrics / Elmer R. Grossman.
        p.   cm.
    ISBN 0–7216–3666–7
    1. Pediatrics.   I. Title.
    [DNLM: 1. Pediatrics.   WS 100 G878e 1994]
RJ45.G85   1994
618.92—dc20
DNLM/DLC   93–13862

International Edition
ISBN   0–7216–5329–4

EVERYDAY PEDIATRICS   ISBN 0–7216–3666–7

Printed in the United States of America

Last digit is the print number: 9   8   7   6   5   4   3   2   1

House calls were still standard when I started practice in Berkeley 33 years ago. One afternoon, early in my career, I went to see a sick patient of one of my partners. The mother opened the door and greeted me happily, "Oh, you must be the new doctor we've heard about. Welcome to the Berkeley Pediatric Group!" Her words made clear that it was somehow her group as much as ours, a collaborative endeavor among the patients, their families, and the staff. And that is what our group has tried to be.

It is to the Berkeley Pediatric Medical Group community that I wish to dedicate this book. My partners, our staff, and our patients have given me a wonderful, supportive, and satisfying place in which to practice medicine, to teach and grow and live.

❧ PREFACE AND ACKNOWLEDGMENTS

This book is written for young clinicians interested in the medical care of children: the pediatricians, family doctors, and nurse practitioners who will be responsible for the new generation. The problems and the opportunities of pediatric practice have changed very little during the four decades since I left medical school. Common diseases are still common, human growth and development proceed along the same lines. Laboratory aids are more powerful and drugs more numerous, but the general rules of medical management are still much the same. The great difference is that clinical teaching is now nearly exclusively in the hands of the medical school specialist, whose approach has become increasingly based on molecular biology and high-tech instrumentation. The relative simplicities of ordinary medical problems are easily overlooked; the patient becomes invisible behind the screen of machines, monitors, and print-outs.

In this book I suggest some of the ways in which everyday well-child and sick-child care can remain small-scale, office-based, low-tech, and simple. I believe that it is possible and desirable to render medical care to children in this fashion. It is a great deal more pleasant for the child and family, less expensive for whoever has to pay for it, and more interesting and satisfying for the practitioner.

The reader will note that these practice-based approaches are sometimes heterodox, if not to say idiosyncratic. I am aware of the danger of mistaking my odd notions based on limited experience for wisdom based on eternal truths. The reader should remain at least as skeptical as the writer.

A few acknowledgments for help with this book are in order: my partners at the Berkeley Pediatric Medical Group, especially Susan D. Ehrlich and Keith C. Quirolo, for critical comments on the work in progress; my wife, for forcing me to shorten sentences and to use correct punctuation and clearer phraseology; and my editors at W.B. Saunders, Lisette Bralow and Judith Fletcher, for guiding me through publication with patience and good humor.

Elmer R. Grossman, M.D.

❧ CONTENTS

Contents

x

❧ CHAPTER 1

What Do You Mean, "Everyday Pediatrics"?

Every time a new partner joins us at the Berkeley Pediatric Group an invariable sequence follows. A clinical problem arises and the newcomer seeks advice about it. The more experienced doctor outlines his or her approach and so elicits the response, "But that doesn't sound like the way they taught us in residency."

The newcomer is correct. We truly do have a different approach in our version of the real world. This book is about my world of private pediatric practice and about the challenges and opportunities that exist in that milieu, which differs in so many ways from the world of teaching hospitals: the patients are different, the diseases are different, the setting is different, and the doctors are different.

Our patients, like those in many offices, are mostly middle-class; a great deal follows from that simple statement. Their families own and use calendars; they live by the clock and in the future; they have settled places of abode, by and large; and they can usually understand and follow instructions. They share, in a general way, the doctor's ideas about the causes and treatments of disease that have become part of the dominant culture of the age. None of these statements is likely to be true of a significant proportion of the patients I see during attending rounds at our local children's hospital or our county hospital.

The diseases encountered in pediatric practice are different. We see our patients early in the course of illnesses, usually before complications have arisen—sometimes too early, in fact. We see the mild forms of serious illness that never reach the hospital or the subspecialist. My diabetic and asthmatic patients very rarely, if ever, are admit-

1

ted. My patients with rheumatoid disease are usually not very sick. Even our anorexics look pretty well nourished most of the time. When our kids get sick, they start from a healthier base, without the pre-existing problems of iron deficiency, untreated parasites, and poor eating habits.

The setting of our practice is different in that our families know us and trust us; we don't have to practice defensive medicine and we don't have to sell ourselves; nor do we have a hierarchy of senior physicians looking over our shoulders, awaiting the opportunity to criticize us for having omitted ordering an axillary cobalt or a serum rhubarb. Of course, neither do we have a reassuring senior resident or experienced professor handy to protect us and our patients from our mistakes.

The doctors in our practice are different. A primary care pediatrician learns to look for patterns of illness, rather than use algorithms. We learn to expect the common diseases; our differential diagnosis lists are short; and we expect our patients to get better. Eventually, we become fairly deliberate; sometimes we can sit back and wait for the diagnosis to declare itself. It does not always need to be wrested from the patient by lab analysis. In contrast, the hospital-based subspecialist is schooled by an experience of severe illness, uncommon problems, nasty complications as a matter of course, much more urgency, and today, the utilization committee urging him to discharge the patient "yesterday."

Because medical school and residency teaching are now firmly in the hands of subspecialists, the new graduates imbibe their approach. A considerable amount of re-education has to take place when primary care pediatrics outside the teaching hospital is undertaken.

This means that we must learn from our own practice. However, we all know how unreliable and hazardous it is to leap from the uncontrolled experience with a few patients to general conclusions. *Post hoc, ergo propter hoc* is the dangerous trap into which our forefathers in medicine fell for centuries. How can one perform controlled experiments on a miscellany of patients? Well, all that is true enough; yet one does learn in practice. One gains experience, and through close observation, thought, comparison of patients, and search for patterns, one may begin to see some of the subtleties that are lost in the big studies. One develops a critical sense about what is likely and what is possible. In time, one sees fads come and go in medicine. The popularity of the new drug that is the greatest thing since sliced bread eventually fades, and the exciting new test turns out to be a bust. "The book says . . . ," but the book is wrong. Finally, one begins to trust oneself a bit more, not too much, but enough, and becomes an experienced physician.

That is part of what this book is about. I want to share some of what I have learned about practice, not all of which is in the books. There is no pretense of all-inclusiveness; a good deal of what I have to say will be somewhat heterodox and personal, not to say idiosyncratic. The purposes are to offer pragmatic advice—especially about topics often ignored during training, to point out some possibilities in practice, and to stimulate argument and thought in the reader.

Of course, a dash of skepticism is appropriate. As I mentioned, my experience is largely based on a practice in Berkeley, California, a wonderful little city but hardly middle America. The reader's place of practice may provide constraints very different from those of the free-wheeling Bay Area. The other ingredients in my professional life have included practice at an Air Force base, a brief stint with Permanente Medical Group at the small Kaiser Hospital in southern California, and a lot of hospital teaching. Since 1959, I've taught at the University of California in San Francisco; attending rounds at Moffitt Hospital and San Francisco General Hospital have provided a corrective to Berkeley parochialism. Attending at our local Children's Hospital in Oakland has given me a look at practices of my colleagues in the East Bay; the settings range from affluent suburbia to the ghetto and barrios of Oakland. In short, I have a fair idea of the variety of subcultures served by pediatricians in other areas, but most of what I've learned in office practice is influenced by the academic and liberal setting of our college town. The reader will, doubtless, modify to suit.

❧ CHAPTER 2
The Possibilities of Practice

How will you define your life in medicine? The question may seem grandiose, but it isn't. It is precisely the question you answer when you decide where and with whom to practice. It would be a pity to arrive at the answer without carefully considering the problem, and that is the subject of this chapter.

To a considerable degree, your place of practice defines its possibilities. What is expected of the pediatrician, the family doctor, or the nurse practitioner? Each community has a set of standards, more accurately, each has *sets* of standards, because there are always a variety of social circles within every town or city, and each has its own characteristics. In our group practice we notice that wealthy families use our services very selectively; they call us about illnesses only when they are clearly in trouble: "He's had a 104° fever for 5 days, so we thought we'd better call." Our middle-class families are much more likely to call early. The well-to-do also tend to use much less well-child care; their message seems to be, "We are comfortably in charge here, thank you, and we'll let you know when we want you." The middle-class families are the easiest to work with; they generally share our understanding of illness, and they are (more or less) willing to accept advice. In our community they want and expect attention to their concerns about the growth and development of their children, as well as answers to their questions about disease or injury. The expectations of our poor parents are not so glibly categorized, because they are such a varied lot. Some are counterculture families who use us with considerable wariness when the homeopathic remedies don't seem to be working. Some are working poor who are delighted to have doctors who treat them with respect and who would be happy to cooperate in our treatment plans if their finances and their general mode of existence allowed it. Unfortunately, they don't live by the calendar, and long-term care is spotty. The expectations of our welfare families are formed by their past experience with the medical community; they have generally been patients in county hospitals and clinics, and they are inured to anonymous, hurried, and not necessarily gentle encounters. We have a hard time convincing them that it is worthwhile for them to come to appointments on time, or to come at all; they drift back to emergency room care, especially on nights and weekends; the likelihood of compliance with medical advice is remote.

Ethnic and religious groups also have wonderfully varied ideas about appropriate medical care. Some of my families are ex–Christian Scientists; they have a terrible time using medical care at all. At the other extreme are Jewish families for whom medical care is a central support for existence; being Jewish myself, I know how they feel, but at times I wish we were not quite so intense about it. (The late anthropologist Mark Zborowski did a great study of ethnic differences in patient behavior. He spent several years at a Veterans Administration hospital observing patients of Italian, Irish, Jewish, and "Old American" stock and found a striking variation in how patients perceived their illnesses, symptoms, medical attendants and treatment. The Old Americans ignored symptoms and put off seeking care, but they were cooperative and uncomplaining when they became patients. The staff found them easiest to work with. The Irish were vague about symptoms, accepted their care passively, and were pessimistic about their medical problems. The Italians sought care earlier and complained a lot about pain; they did not have to be stoic. The Jews could also express pain freely; they were the patients most anxious and most eager for a diagnosis, as distinct from wanting relief from symptoms. (They also were the most critical of the medical care they received.) Our northern California practice brings us into contact with many Latinos, Asians, and Pacific Islanders. Every one of these groups has a specific medical subculture with strongly held beliefs, most of which will be unknown to their medical advisers. If grandma at home thinks your prescription fails to fit the criteria of the subculture, grandma's ideas are likely to supersede yours.

Of course, some communities have such obvious medical needs that personal preferences of either doctors or patients are overridden.

When pediatricians began to move into the small towns around here a few decades ago, the pressing requirement was for the care of acute, severe illness. The niceties of well-child supervision had to wait. Now, however, practitioners in many areas can develop subspecialty interests as part of a general pediatric practice. This is especially easy to do if one is part of a group, because intragroup referrals are available. For a solo practitioner, getting referrals from one's colleagues is difficult, because the other pediatricians in town fear the loss of the patient; it is safer to refer to a distant (and inconvenient) consultant.

The remaining big question is this: What do you hope to accomplish during your 30 or 40 years of practice? This omnibus question includes what you want for yourself, how you want to live your life with your family, what the family needs, how much money you hope to earn, and how hard you want to work. It also includes what you want to do for your patients, your medical community, and the town or city where you will live. As you become acquainted with people in a new place, a thousand opportunities will present themselves for service to hospitals, the medical society, community clubs, religious groups, schools, youth groups—all the volunteer organizations that constitute much of the structure of American society. I remember vividly the words of a senior doctor as he explained the need for involvement: "An organization is like a tapestry which is always wearing and fraying; it needs continual mending and reweaving." You will discover that your status as a physician gives you an automatic position of respect, which you may feel you don't really deserve. After all those years at the bottom of the medical ladder, it is something of a shock to find that people pay attention to you.

The defining truth for most of us, in choosing the forms of our careers, is that we can't do everything. Some of my teachers in medical school looked like "Super Docs" to me. They seemed to have time and skill and energy for absolutely everything one could imagine doing. Our professor of anatomy, for example, was also a prize-winning painter, boxer, sailor, champion golfer, medievalist, historian, orthopedic surgeon, and researcher. There were many others like him, and they certainly set a standard for the level of achievement one should aspire to. Well, I've slowly come to understand that this standard is unrealistic. One must discover the size of one's own talent and strength; it is a waste of time comparing oneself to Einstein, Cushing, or Osler. It is also a mistake to compare one's income to that of surgeons, anesthesiologists, or anyone else in medicine. When we chose general practice or pediatrics we didn't take vows of poverty, but we certainly had noticed that these are not roads to affluence. Expect to feel a bit greedy and jealous at times, expect to drive a smaller car, and remember that you are still in the highest 5% or so of American incomes.

During the early years of practice, the need to develop and experience a sense of competence fuels the effort of long hours of work. It is a heady and exciting time, and the balance of interest and focus often favors professional growth over family and self. I think this is the most dangerous time for marriages. Everybody is too busy, and the needs of the marriage relationship are easily forgotten. The story is the same in the families of other young professionals or business people; we aren't unique, but maybe our situations are a little bit worse than others'. Perhaps this is because we have defined ourselves as people who attend to other people's problems. We tend to avoid and deny our own human needs: "I'm fine—you are the patient." It is also the time when we are likely to have young children of our own. Ask the grown kids of doctors if they saw enough of dad or mom; their answers will depress you and possibly change the balance you find for your own family. Making time for oneself is an idea that some doctors never do stumble over. But, if you don't spend some intelligence and energy in the care and nurturing of yourself as a person, a certain narrowness may be the cost. Not long ago I met an old medical friend who had left practice the previous year, and asked, "How do you like retirement?" He grimaced and replied, "It's just awful, Elmer. Don't ever do it." There had never been time for anything in his life except his beloved medicine, and now there was nothing in his life. You will notice that I'm talking about only the *problems* of balance in one's life; I've offered no solutions at all. That's because I don't know what you need or how you might attain it. This chapter is a crude navigation map with hints about the dangerous shoals and reefs; we all have to find our own harbors.

In the last chapter I'll ask you to look at a different set of opportunities: teaching, writing, and research in practice. These all can be exciting and great fun, but they are frosting on the cake and not how you will make your living. Those practical organizational and economic questions are the subject of the next chapter.

CHAPTER 3
Organizing Your Work

Because I joined an ongoing group practice after I left residency, I was spared the task of learning how the business of medicine is accomplished. Someone already knew how to order stationery and send out bills, find the best supplier for 2 × 2s, hire staff, and handle the rest of the everyday mechanics of a practice. Over the years I've learned something about these issues, because we take yearly turns at being the group's business manager. However, the truth is that there are better sources of information than me. Books have been written on the business aspects of medicine; if you are starting out on your own, buy one. What I want to talk about in this chapter is the organization of the medical side of your practice: who will do what; how long it will take; where and how it will be done.

Who Does What

This innocent little phrase goes to the heart of our work. In a busy practice there is always too much to do, too many people to see, too much information to convey. So "who does what" implies the need for decisions about what work is important for the clinician to do and what can be delegated. Years ago a new combined diphtheria, pertussis, tetanus (DPT) and polio vaccine was developed, and I asked my old chief of pediatrics what he thought of the advance. "It's awful," he said. When I responded with surprise, he explained that giving the immunization shots was the center and purpose of the well-child visit, as far as he was concerned. He never let anyone else

9

in his office give injections, and if there were fewer shots to give, he believed that his role was diminished. In my office, on the other hand, I practically never give injections, but I try to keep a monopoly on the dispensing of medical information.

This starts at the front desk. Our receptionists have a multiplicity of tasks, all of them crucial to the functioning of the establishment. They provide a first impression of the Berkeley Pediatric Medical Group to new patients and give information about the office, about which insurance plans we deal with, about the doctors—who is female, who is male, who is new, and who is not new. They relay hundreds of messages from patients, doctors, labs, and hospitals. They turn away calls from stock and bond salesmen (don't those folks understand how little money pediatricians make?), drug company representatives, insurance salespeople. Most important, they decide which call requires an appointment that day, which pain justifies an immediate visit, which anxious parent is put through to the doctor. They develop an ear for the complex problem that will not fit into a 10- or 15-minute illness-visit time slot. All of this must be done while sitting in a noisy anteroom next to the well-child waiting room, listening to small children rolling the wooden trucks down the slide ("No, Johnny, the slide is for people, not trucks"). There is a constant stream of doctors, nurses, and business office people coming and going behind them, who are looking for charts, lab reports, and telephone message lists. There is also a stream of patients asking for new appointments, taxi service, information about billing, forms to be completed, and prescriptions to be telephoned in ("What's the name of that pharmacy—the big pink one at the corner of Telegraph and— what is that cross-street?"). There are doctors asking, for example, that the lady on line 6 be given an appointment this morning and "Would you please ask the Children's Hospital lab *where is that report?*" They stay pretty busy. However, they do not give medical advice more complex than "Give him sips of ginger ale every few minutes until the doctor calls you back." We don't want them to take medical responsibility; they are neither doctors nor nurses, and we want everybody to understand whose job is what. This means that the doctors handle a large load of telephone calls about quite trivial and mundane matters. Needless to say, on a busy day during an influenza outbreak, questions about an old and recalcitrant diaper rash are not wholly welcome, but that is the price we pay for keeping medical advice-giving in our own hands.

Now, you may be wondering why we don't have an advice nurse or a nurse practitioner, as every other progressive office does. Why don't we save our valuable medical time for valuable medical matters? The reasons are multiple. First, the six of us would have a hard time agreeing even on routine advice. One of the joys of the way we work is that each doctor can proceed in the way that is most comfortable for her or him, without having to follow a cook-book consensus of the partners. For example, I have never been convinced that limiting lactose is necessary in the treatment of ordinary gastroenteritis, so I recommend a dilute formula or milk early in the disease. My partners usually proscribe milk for the first days of diarrhea, which is a little confusing to the patients who get divergent advice if they call at different times. That is fine with me; I think it is realistic and healthy for our families to know that doctors disagree (hardly a new idea!). I like our flexibility.

The second reason for keeping medical advice in medical hands is safety. The risk of mismanaging a situation with unwise telephone advice is always with us. Over the years, one becomes pretty skilled at what Theodore Reik called "listening with the third ear." He was talking about the psychotherapeutic situation, but it applies to general medicine, too. One becomes sensitized to the meaning of patterns and nuances in what is being said; I'd rather have that listening done by a doctor.

The third reason is probably the most important one. The more often I talk with a family, the better we get to know each other and the closer we can become. I want them to think of me—not the group or the advice nurse—as their primary source of pedatric advice. The disadvantages are the increased demands on my time and patience and the probability that a rather dependent relationship will be fostered with some families. The advantage is that they will think of asking me for help with or opinions about the many problems that will arise in their lives as families. I can be helpful only if I know they need help, and I want to encourage that expectation.

It is clear, then, that the role of the nurses in our office is rather circumscribed. They weigh and measure the kids, test eyes and ears, give shots, cleanse wounds, and do dressings. When children come in for illness visits they take a mini-history to alert the doctor to the general problem area (and to find out what clothes will likely need to come off). They are supposed to take temperatures of sick kids, and this often evolves into an interesting tug-of-war with the parent. The nurse asks, "Does he have a fever?" The parent answers (rapidly applying fingers to child's forehead), "No." The nurse responds, "The doctor always wants a measured temperature, so let's take his diaper off." The parent rejoins, "Oh, he really hates having his temperature taken." What happens next depends on the balance of forces: the nurse's guess about how annoyed the doctor will be at the absence of a real measurement, the parent's guess about how long it will take to return the child to a calm state after the expected struggle, and the child's understanding that the adults are unsure of how to proceed.

Despite the limited range of nurse-parent-child interactions, a warm and deep affection develops among the families and the nurses, who tend to stay with us for many years. As they come to know the families, the nurses are frequently sources of information for us, especially about the emotional state of a child or a parent whom we are going to see. On the other hand, their role in giving advice to parents is limited. The one exception is in the management of home phototherapy. During the past 2 decades we have treated a couple of hundred jaundiced infants with phototherapy at home. During most of that time the nurses have been in charge of the entire procedure. They set up the lights, arrange for an appropriate home environment, teach the family how to manage the treatment and how to keep the needed records, and make daily home visits to oversee everything. The doctor keeps in touch by telephone and through the nurse and usually makes a house call as well, but the main task is the nurse's responsibility. It works beautifully.

Within the framework of a pediatric practice, teaching and giving information can be accomplished in a number of ways besides the Mark Hopkins method of the teacher on one end of a log and the student on the other. We have experimented with night meetings for groups of parents to talk about particular topics in child-rearing and a Saturday morning group for adolescents to discuss their concerns. We gave up the parent groups because of doctor fatigue; the adolescent groups were stopped because of teenage resistance. We make use of information boards in the waiting room; often there is a parent reading something about safety, immunizations, or available community services. Printed hand-out literature on a variety of topics is a great help. The topics include allergy, nutrition, safety, acne, and various book lists. We have written some of these ourselves; some are pirated from others; and some are provided by health organizations. We stay away from commercial publications, preferring to avoid the implied endorsement of a product.

Underlying all of this information-giving activity is the general set of largely unspoken premises of our practice. We seem to have decided that pediatrics should be prevention-oriented, and that means investing a lot of time providing well-child care, explaining why we do what we do with illness, attempting to involve the families in sharing responsibility in medical decisions rather than pretending that *ex cathedra* pronouncements are sufficient, and trying to build the families' abilities to cope with the problems of their children in health and in illness. This is a tall order. It follows that one must spend a good bit of time with each patient contact, whether in the office, the hospital, the home, or over the telephone. A pediatrician in another office in town was recently complaining to me about one of his partners who always had long telephone lists, which he considered a waste and a mistake. *His* patients, he said, had learned not to call him with unnecessary questions. I envied him his short telephone lists, but I don't know a better way of approaching my rather different goals than by being available and taking time.

Listen to what people say about our profession. They complain that they wait 50 minutes in the office and are rewarded with a 5-minute visit. They say that the doctor comes to the hospital, hardly comes into the room, and is gone before they know it. The message is, "I'm the Doctor and my time is important." Well, so we are and so it is, but their time is important too. What follows is the decision to honor their needs as well as one's own.

Grossman's First Law of Medical Time: If you are chronically late, your schedule is not realistic. Ask yourself why. Are you deliberately late to one-up the patient? "I can make you wait for me" is a nasty but effective show of power. Is it just wishful thinking? "That family isn't really all that difficult; I'm sure a 15-minute appointment will suffice to check her acne, her migraine, and her school problems."

Grossman's Second Law of Medical Time: Two kids take longer

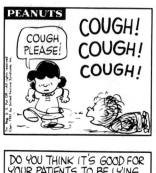
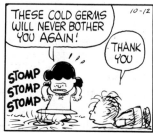
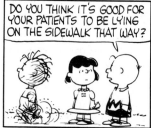
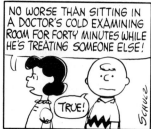

Courtesy of United Features Syndicate, Inc.

than one kid. When the mother asks, "By the way, since we are here, could you take a look at _____," you have an opportunity to be a Nice Guy (the occupational disease of pediatricians) and take the requested look. If you do, you will then be 15 minutes later for the rest of the day. You will also have taught that mother to repeat the request whenever it is convenient for the next 20 years. Alternatively, you have the opportunity to make the point that seeing the second child means that everybody else would have to wait that much longer and that you'd hate to inconvenience all those widows and orphans in the waiting room. This is remarkably difficult to do without coming across as a prissy nerd, but it may be worth a try. What I often say is "Let me see if my next patient is waiting; if not, I'll be happy to see _____." If the next patient is already chafing at the bit, I suggest that I can see the child sometime later.

Grossman's Third Law of Medical Time: My time is not your time. Every doctor discovers the pace that passeth understanding, that is to say, how long it takes one to accomplish the particular task. When I started practice, I noted that each of my partners had quite different schedules for well-child and sick-child visits. Trial and error were required for my discovery of a pattern that suited me. I need about 30 to 40 minutes for the first hospital visit for a newborn, even more if it is the only hospital visit I'll have with that mother; a house call to a newborn takes me 45 minutes plus travel time; a new patient workup takes at least 1 hour; a routine well-child visit takes at least 30 minutes; most routine illness visits take 15 minutes. A quick return visit, typically for otitis, requires only 10 minutes. For teenagers' checkups, I schedule 30 minutes for the patient and 15 to 30 minutes on another day for the parent. Discussion visits usually take 45 to 60 minutes, whether for diet counseling, allergy control planning, or psychological problems.

This brings us to **Grossman's Fourth Law of Medical Time: Happiness is a reasonable work load.** If I have scheduled my time rationally and I stay more or less on schedule, I love my work. When I allow my schedule to become too crowded and I am rushed and late, I hate my work, resent my patients, and wonder why anyone would ever choose to be a pediatrician.

The questions to be asked of all law-makers are pertinent here: (1) Do you really expect people to follow these rules? (2) Do you follow them yourself? The obvious answers are (1) No and (2) No. These are hints, rather than commandments. I am sure that I am a happier person and a better pediatrician when I give them more than lip service; perhaps the same will be true for you.

❧ CHAPTER 4

Patient-Doctor Relationships in Pediatrics

One of the interesting aspects of pediatric practice is the wonderful multiplicity of doctor-patient relationships. If you have the good fortune to start with a prenatal visit, you are instantly aware that the entire family is your patient; you will have some sort of professional relationship with everyone at home and often with distant family members as well. This comes as a surprise only because of the notion that the human being is the unit of human existence, a widely held illusion based on the misleading fact that our skins separate us from the rest of the world. However, we are not much more separate as individuals than sponges in a colony or bees in a hive, so intimately are we linked to one another. You meet the pregnant woman, and perhaps the father, and become involved in family issues about child care, return to work, help with the infant; you are also concerned about the mother's health, drug history, and plans to nurse. The views of the father must be attended to—how does he feel about the baby, nursing, and the imminent change in his family life? How will the newcomer affect the existence of the other kids? At this stage in your pediatric relationship, the least important family member is probably the unborn infant.

This confusion continues after the baby is born and at home. You discover that the obstetrician has lost interest in the mother about 10 minutes post partum. Only rarely will the mother have been given adequate information about her needs for rest and food; no one will have raised questions about the new family's needs for support and for a little peace and quiet. If the mother is nursing, you are usually safe in assuming that information about the process has been limited to a few commercial hand-outs and the automatic prescription of a totally useless nipple cream. When problems with nursing arise, the mother may find it difficult to decide where to turn for help, and even harder to obtain worthwhile advice.

Are you convinced? My point is that the family is your patient, which is fine, although spheres of influence and areas of authority may be unclear. You have to avoid stepping on the toes of other doctors, but you also have to be sure that the medical needs of the family are somehow being met.

The most obvious patient-pediatrician relationship in the new-born period is with the mother. Yes, I know that newborns are sentient beings and without doubt share your eagerness to begin a long and fruitful relationship with you as the doctor, but pragmatically, the mother and her needs bulk larger. The isolation of so many nuclear families is an immense problem for new mothers; often they are exhausted, unsure, and anxious, meeting new situations minute by minute, and generally about as needy as you can imagine. If you give them a willing ear for their problems, a truly useful bond can be made. There is, of course, the built-in hazard of fostering a dependency that is in no one's best interest. I don't know how to avoid this except by developing a pattern of encouraging the parents to examine their alternatives and reach their own conclusions. That is, in any case, the best way to proceed with most medical advice. We physicians see dramatic examples of interventionist medicine during every stage of our training. The unconscious victim of an automobile accident, the child with meningitis, or the surgical patient with an uncontrolled bleeder requires us to make the necessary and lifesaving decisions. As models for deciding how to manage a wakeful infant, the emergency room and the surgical suite are a bit off the mark, but the old habits of authoritarian activism are comfortable, ego-satisfying, and hard to shake.

So where does that leave us with the mother? She needs medical advice and emotional support. She needs to lean on you at times, but in the long run she needs to feel her own competence and strength. If you care about her family, you can show it by following up on illnesses, making unsolicited telephone call-backs on problems, and being reachable when needed. You will have some families in your practice for whom these niceties will be hard to manage. I know that

I find it very difficult to decide to call the mother who always finds my suggestions untenable and who always has a list of whining complaints that she wants me to cure. Perhaps if I were a Better Person, I would have learned to welcome these opportunities for service, but I'm not. I have been known to hang up abruptly, for which I hope the Academy of Pediatrics forgives me.

The father is a newly emerging figure in the pediatrician's office. When I started in practice, the presence of a male parent was an aberration and always rather startling. I could tell myself that I felt discomfort with fathers because it was easier to communicate with mothers; they knew what was happening and the fathers did not. This was, and is, true; it is also beside the point. The reality was simply my lack of experience. I can't tell you how to communicate with parents of either gender, but whenever you can, stand back and observe the differences in the doctor-parent relationships. This is partly a function of the differing sexual roles in our culture. I watch my female partners develop a kind of collegiality with the mothers in their practices; it looks wonderfully comfortable. Male doctors' relationships with mothers are inevitably colored by the one-up position of males in American society; both parties to the encounter may expect more power to be in the hands of the male. In our community, at any rate, this is by no means always acceded to by the female, but the stage is set in this manner.

There is also the possibility of some sexual tension between the doctor and parent; both are presumably sexually mature adults, and the situation is sometimes physically intimate and often emotionally labile. Added to this may be the halo effect of some hero worship on the part of the parent; the doctor may need a firm grasp of the Hippocratic Oath to stay in a purely medical mode.

As fathers have taken a larger role in child-rearing, I have gradually become used to them. As a group, they really are unsure of their medical role. They don't know much about the details of illness care, and their knowledge about everyday routines is usually incomplete. Because men use medical care much less often than women do and because many fathers have never learned home nursing skills, they may be less competent in carrying out medical advice. Add to this a dash of male-to-male competitiveness, and the average father and the average male pediatrician do not have the most comfortable and reliable collaboration. The doctor says, "I see that Sam didn't come back for a recheck on his ear infection." The mother responds, "Oh, his father must have brought him in for that illness. He didn't tell me you needed to see Sam again." There is no solution, but you might make a point of writing your instructions and hope that dad shows the paper to mom.

When families are young, vulnerable, and needy, the parents can develop a troubling amount of dependence on the pediatrician. The absence of extended families as sources of trusted advice and support, the multiplicity of competing and contradictory "experts" in the media, the rapid changes in child-rearing styles—all these factors leave new parents confused at a time when they want to feel safe and competent. For a few years they may lean heavily on a reliable doctor. I don't see this as such a bad thing, especially if it is temporary, as it usually is. After a while most families develop a sense of their ability to cope with problems on their own. A good sign is the gradual drop-off in telephone questions and the eventual lessening of interest in well-child care. When I first noticed this pattern in my practice, my feelings were hurt; didn't they want my help anymore? Now I see it as success; after all, if the doctor has done an adequate job, the parents ought to be able to fly solo most of the time.

When I first started working with children during medical school, I'd observe the easy comfort of the experienced nurses and doctors working with kids from the newborn nursery to the adolescent ward. They had obviously mastered relational skills that I hadn't even heard about. But, in time, even the psychologically obtuse student begins to learn what works with the child patient. Sometimes it is the little trick of letting the fussy infant suck on one's finger during the exam or that of cuing the baby's smiling response with one's own smiling face and nodding head. One learns to make eye contact when the child is interested and to avoid it when the child is fearful. What I've observed by watching other practitioners is that many different styles of interaction are acceptable; the way you act with children can't be legislated, because it follows from your personality. If you are "soft-and-fuzzy," that's how you will be with kids; if you are not, you won't be. In any case, the child eventually responds to your ease and competence. It is a fine accomplishment to be able to pick up and comfort a fussing infant and to be able to listen to and reassure a miserable and frantic teenager.

The child also learns about you from the parents. Their message to the child really defines the child's expectations of the doctor. How many times I have heard a parent say to the sick and frightened child, "It's all right; the doctor will make you better." What an incredibly powerful statement! My mother and father, the source of everything in my life, the embodiment of strength, have brought me to this magician who will take away my pain! I think this is an important component of the life-long reverence and respect that we enjoy in our role as doctors and that we feel toward our doctors when we ourselves are patients.

The child's response to the doctor naturally changes as the child grows. The infant is usually interested in you as another friendly adult, at least until the middle of the first year when stranger anxiety appears. From then until age 2 or 3 years, you may be perceived as the embodiment of evil; it isn't your fault and it will pass. The small child's distaste for us makes perfect sense. After all, the medical encounter is absolutely peculiar and nonsensical in relation to the rest of the child's life. The child is taken to an unclassifiable environment, stripped unceremoniously of clothing, weighed, measured, poked, and prodded by solemn grownups. Why should they like us? This anxiety can be mitigated to some extent; the office can be made to appear somewhat homelike, the staff can wear ordinary clothes, and the child can be provided with playthings.

By the toddler stage, one can increasingly direct one's social attention and speech to the child. I like to ask even 3- and 4-year-olds about symptoms, about which ear I should look in first, and about nursery school and playmates. I don't learn much, but I am showing the child that I am his or her doctor and that I am interested in what the child's experience might be. By middle childhood, the child is contributing substantially to the encounter, often contradicting the parent's report.

Balancing the continuing relationship with the parents while developing the relationship with the child is a nice trick. During well-child visits from the age of 3 years and onward, I try to send the child out of the examining room to play or to complete nursing procedures such as vision tests; this allows some private time for discussion of topics the parent may want to keep from the child. It is instructive to watch the interaction of parent and child as this brief separation is attempted; one learns a great deal about the parent's ability to set limits and the child's willingness to cooperate in a situation perceived as challenging.

When the child enters early adolescence, I ask the families to split wellness-care visits: a full appointment for the teenager alone and a briefer appointment for the parents on another day. One gauges the timing of this change by the adolescent's maturity: it is usually appropriate at about 13 years of age for either boys or girls, although some girls may need mother's presence until 14 or 15 years of age. It is fascinating that some mothers have difficulty separating even at later ages. I have a few families with college-age kids whose mothers still accompany them for medical visits.

How do you manage your teenage patients? They are a varied lot, and no simple recipe suffices. Perhaps the first point is to become aware of our own problems with this age group. We may find ourselves identifying so powerfully with them that our medical judgment is clouded. I must say that this is a greater danger for the young doctor than for people of my age, who are more likely to identify with the parents. From the adolescent's point of view, we probably are most often seen as another part of the adult power structure, perhaps as the agents of the parents. However, some adolescents take us seriously, use us as role models, and heed what we say. As I hear and read about what various experts say I should accomplish with my adolescent patients (establish a trusting and mutually respectful relationship, elicit emotional and physical concerns, provide guidance regarding drugs, sex, diet, exercise, body care, and so on), I feel guilty and inadequate until I stop to consider the reality of doing all this. So, play it loose, try to find out what they need, and be honest about what you know and what you don't know.

A few paragraphs ago I mentioned that I have trouble being civil, let alone helpful, to certain mothers. This is part of a larger issue: how do you respond to patients (children, teenagers, or parents) who you really don't like? There is no point to pretending that you will like all of the people in your practice; you won't and you shouldn't. Sometimes you will have good and sufficient reasons for finding a patient undesirable. There will be families who fail to keep appointments, ignore medical advice, tell you lies, leave their medical bills unpaid, or commit similar felonies. There will also be families with whom you are just not simpatico. A safe assumption is that they are not particularly fond of you, either. In any of these cases you have the choice of bringing the problem to the attention of a parent so that some conscious choice can be made. You all may be happier apart.

Finally, a word should be said about pediatric grandchildren. When your patients become parents and bring their children to you for medical care, you will have a most satisfying experience that brings a certain sense of validation: after all the unpleasant things you had to do to this person, she still trusts you to take care of her baby. More important, there is a sense of continuity. Recently, a grandmother was sitting in our waiting room while her grandchild was seeing one of my partners. She looked around appraisingly and commented that she had been coming to our office in one role or another for 40 years. It was a lovely statement to hear.

❧ CHAPTER 5

Get-Acquainted Visits and Prenatal Visits

When a family of mine moves to a distant city, parents often ask me how to find a new pediatrician. My advice is to ask as many people as possible about their own doctors, to find a clinical faculty person if there is a nearby medical school, and to arrange a get-acquainted visit with the most likely candidate. I am aware that some doctors resent and refuse these "I'm going to look you over" sessions, but there is much to commend in them. They give parents a useful impression of you and your practice, and they let you set the stage for the kind of patient-doctor relationship that you wish to establish. I use them to arrange for the transfer of medical records, explain our use of well-child visits, and discuss the necessity of new-patient checkup appointments. What I want to avoid is the hurriedly arranged first illness visit that involves a complex set of old problems needing extra time to unravel. A brief get-acquainted visit can keep this from happening.

Prenatal visits are a special get-acquainted opportunity. From the pediatrician's point of view, a visit with the expectant parents is solid gold. In a practice that looks forward to decades of contact with families, a base of invaluable information can be laid and a sense of the parents can be developed that will inform one's efforts for many years. I want to know as much as I can about these people: who they are, where they come from, where they were educated, and what they do for a living. What about health problems, heritable and otherwise? I ask about the family religion, because there are substantial differences in the medical expectations of the various faiths. How the family perceives the medical establishment in general, and doctors in particu-

25

lar, will become clear as the parents talk. The more explicitly these feelings are stated, the better the outcome will be for us all. In fact, some of my most useful prenatal visits have concluded with my suggestion to the family that they consider seeing another doctor, because what they needed, wanted, and expected wasn't going to happen with me.

The areas of concern that parents expect you to ask about are the "medical"matters of the pregnancy, and of course one wants the facts: how the pregnancy has progressed, complications, tests, drugs, where the baby will be born, who will attend the birth, what childbirth training has been accomplished, and whether the baby will be nursed or bottle-fed? A lot of information is conveyed in the way the mother answers your question "Do you plan to nurse your baby?" Everyone is in for trouble if she grimaces and says, "I'll try."

Perhaps nothing in the visit is more useful than the impression one gets of the whole family. Does the father come to the visit? If not, why not? How do the two parents interact in the office? Who is in charge of what? Of course, the presence of other children in the family is a central subject: what kinds of kids are they? what do the parents expect of them in relation to the newborn? are there stepchildren or half-siblings somewhere, and what will be their roles in the new baby's life? I'm also interested in the grandparents; I ask about their jobs, their health, their marital status, where they live. If a grandparent is coming to help out after the baby is born, I want to know if the parents think that is a good idea.

The last family issues to explore are time of return to work for the working mother and the general subject of help with the new infant. I never cease to be amazed by the optimistic inaccuracy with which first-time parents approach the task of caring for a new baby.

During all of this information-gathering, the doctor is also teaching, both by the emphasis given to a subject (if it weren't important, you wouldn't spend so much time on it) and by the natural interposition of information. More on this topic later.

From the parents' point of view—well, there are many different kinds of parents, and they all have their own viewpoints. I cannot, in all candor, say that I take delight in the consumerist-model parent who comes equipped with a two-page checklist of questions. For one thing, I don't much like thinking of myself as a commodity to be consumed, a finite part of the Gross Domestic Product, although the notion has a certain cool validity. Perhaps more important, the questions on the checklist are like the lists we all memorized in classes on diagnosis, that is to say, mostly off the mark and a waste of time. I believe that a serious mother asking me where I did my residency does not appreciate the irrelevance of the question to the quality of care I can give her and her child. If she were to ask about my philosophy of practice, the answer would be more rewarding to her and more fun for me.

Most of the parents new to my practice use the visit to get a general sense of our office and our staff, and an overall feeling about what I might be like as their child's doctor. They ask specific questions about the pros and cons of circumcision; they want my views on feeding; and they talk about the anticipated problems with older siblings. There are often questions about fees and insurance. Not infrequently they are doctor-shopping, but they rarely mention it. If they do, I tell them how useful I believe it to be; you might as well start out with a doctor with whom you are comfortable.

How the visit is conducted may be as important as its verbal content; the parents can listen to the music as well as to the words. Have you kept them waiting? Did you apologize or explain if you did? Is the consultation room designed to impress the patients with your exalted status, framed diplomas, big desk, and the like? Does it speak of authority (The Doctor) and subservience (everyone else), or does it invite a partnership between parents and physician? Each of us develops a style of practice that reflects who we truly are as people and as doctors. We can't hide, and I don't think we should even try to. If you need to be an authoritarian, "Daddy (or Mommy) knows best" type, so be it. There are plenty of folks who think that's just fine.

In an interview of this sort the beginner may want to rely on a checklist of points to cover; I think that is a mistake. Sticking to an outline may prevent you from following the stream of developing information that can flow from a more conversational approach. Missed information can be obtained at a subsequent visit.

I noted earlier that the processes of learning and teaching are inevitably intertwined. The family history of allergy leads naturally to teaching about the utility of breast-feeding and late introduction of solids to decrease the risk of allergy in the baby. Asking about nursing can lead to instructions about nipple preparation. Questions about the mother's return to work can be followed by comments on the problems of early day care. Part of the teaching is best accomplished with written material, either preprinted or written out on the spot. Recall of medical information imparted orally is abysmal. **Grossman's First Law of Medical Information: If you want it remembered, write it down.** There is no reason to be sanguine about the likelihood that your written words will ever be consulted again, but there is at least a chance, especially if you write legibly. The best retention occurs if parents make their own notes, but I find this process agonizingly slow.

The other topics to be covered with new families have to do with the workings of one's particular practice. In our group we give each family a booklet describing how we think they can best use our services. It explains our goals as doctors, how the practice is organized, when to call, what the office hours are, and how our services are paid for. Some people actually read it.

I generally end the visit with an invitation to telephone if any further issues arise before the baby comes; there are few such calls.

Should one charge for these consultations? In general, I like the idea of free prenatal visits. It gives families more freedom in choosing a pediatrician, and the better their choices are, the happier we all will be. After all, amortizing the lost income for a 30-minute visit over the decades of medical care we hope to provide to a family seems like a small investment. Exceptions do occur. I'll charge for a prenatal when the family wants to see multiple members of our group; there is a limit to how much time we will give away. If I am asked to provide care limited to the newborn period only, I'll charge. If the family has a health insurance plan that habitually underpays me, I charge for the prenatal visit with a wonderful sense of "Gotcha this time!"

Is the scope of material to be talked about daunting? If so, I have misled you. Not every prenatal visit covers every topic; you can pick up any loose threads later. However, one does need enough time; I schedule half an hour and often run a bit over, especially if I am enjoying getting to know new parents. The experience of being allowed into the family through the process of a prenatal visit is a privilege and a joy; don't rush it.

CHAPTER 6

General Issues in Wellness Care

How did we get into the wellness-care business, anyway? When you stop to think about it, there is nothing inevitable about the connection of well-child care with pediatric practice. In many parts of the world, asking the doctor about feeding, growth, developments, and general well-child supervision will be rewarded with puzzled silence or off-handed dismissal. The healthy child isn't supposed to be the doctor's concern. In this part of the world, however, these issues are within the doctor's purview. The questions that arise in wellness care are logically related to ordinary medicine. After all, if the doctor is con-sulted about diet during disease, why not about diet during health? If the doctor is asked about urinary tract infections, why not about enuresis? Added to this connection are two other distinctly American factors: our faith in science as the fount of wisdom and our loss of available grandparents and other stable family sources of information about raising children.

The problem here is the discrepancy between the doctor's old role as dispenser of medical advice and the new role of expert on the care and feeding of children. As the source of information on disease, the doctor presumably knows much more than the patient does and has some objectivity as an observer of the process of disease from which the patient is suffering. Both patient and physician agree that the doctor is an authority, although the fact that doctors disagree is widely understood. As a source of information that addresses the ordinary concerns of parents raising their children, the doctor is on much shakier ground. For one thing, not much is known about child development; it is a new and very soft science. For another, most

29

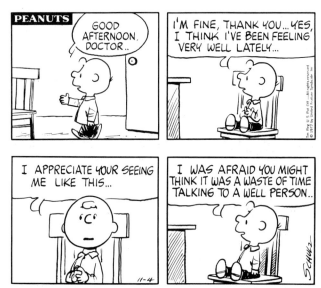

Courtesy of United Features Syndicate, Inc.

doctors are largely unfamiliar with what little firm information is actually available. Our training programs give little attention to well-child care. At least until we have experience with children in our own families, our understanding is likely to be thinly academic at best, supplemented neither by sound science nor by well-digested practical wisdom. One of my partners commented that she still blushes when she remembers the advice she gave in the years before she became a mother herself. To make matters even worse, the doctor's views are often no more than the ordinary prejudices of his or her age, sex, and social class. When I am consulted by a teenager about the treatment of disorders of menstruation, I draw on clinical science; when the same adolescent asks about contraception, my answers are likely to vary with my religion, my age, whether I have teenage children myself, and whether any of them has ever gotten pregnant.

Even if we all were comfortable masters of a well-established academic field of well-child care and even if we all were experienced with the knowledge that may flow from raising our own children, our authority as advice-givers in well-child matters would be limited. That is because the choices we make as parents depend on our personalities and on the goals we have for our children. I was once impressed by a Stanford University study, which indicated that a small child's freedom to explore ideas was enhanced by being reared in a relatively nonrestrictive physical environment. The more the toddler had been surrounded by "No," the less intellectually free the child became. The day after I read this paper, I happened to see two families with infants at the beginning of crawling. One family was upwardly mobile black, with a vigorous and intrusive little boy; the other was aristocratic Austrian with an active little girl. With each mother I raised the question of making the house safe for the baby. I mentioned the research that suggested that giving the baby free reign to explore the entire house might be preferable to confining the baby to a smaller space, at least for mental development. Both mothers listened politely, and at their next visits, both told me that they and their husbands had decided that it was important to keep most of the house baby-free, rather than baby-proof. For both couples, maintaining a civilized and adult style of life took precedence over a theoretical advantage to the child's mind. It was a fascinating and humbling experience for me and was the beginning of my learning the limits of advice-giving.

What follows from the foregoing is the necessity to distinguish between the classical medical model of diagnosis and therapy and the wellness-care model of analysis of the problem and exploration of alternative solutions. Let's take the example of the child who has acute blood loss with a resultant iron-deficiency anemia; the diagnosis is straightforward and so is the treatment. The medical model will probably apply very nicely. In contrast, the child who has iron deficiency secondary to a diet of cow's milk and apple juice bottles presents a different problem. In either situation the anemia can be cured with oral ferrous sulfate, but the bottle addict will have a relapse unless changes are made in the diet. Success in making those changes often depends on figuring out why the old diet was allowed and exploring with the parent the ways in which change can occur. Sometimes all that is needed is information about nutrition; sometimes the underlying problem is one of family relationships. I've seen bottle addiction in families in which parents were unable to set limits, in which exhausted mothers used bottles to get the baby through the night so that the mother could sleep, and in which a parent was keeping a child infantilized. You can't change these behaviors with a prescription for iron. What you can do is explore the situation with the parent and try to help the family understand where the problem lies. When the source of the difficulty is understood, the solution may be obvious; otherwise, the doctor's task is to help the family members examine their possibilities. In this situation, both responsibility and authority remain clearly with the family; the doctor becomes a facilitator. The medical model is no longer sufficient.

This changes the doctor-patient relationship in a fundamental way. When I first began to practice well-child care in this fashion, I had the uncomfortable feeling that I was shifting gears back and forth between two different and conflicting modes. If the child was sick in some clearly somatic way, I was the old-fashioned doc, making a diagnosis and prescribing treatment: "Here is the problem; solve it my way." When the problem was one of behavior or development, I was abruptly changed into the neutral explorer of the situation: "Here is the problem; do we all see it in the same fashion? How might you folks deal with it, so that you solve it your way?" One interesting effect of this dichotomy has been to make it easier for me to share authority in "medical" matters as well. In the long run, we need to admit that most problems of health and disease rest in the hands of the patients rather than the medical profession. Sometimes this is obvious: Do I choose to smoke cigarettes or not? Sometimes it's a little more complicated. My friend Walter needed his damaged heart valves replaced last year. His surgeon gave him the choice of mechanical prostheses, with an increased risk of strokes, or pig valves, with the likelihood of wearing out sooner. It is a nice example of a doctor understanding that the patient has a stake in choosing the treatment and its risks.

Our patients and their parents also have a right to choose. Do we treat this ear infection, with the attendant risk of adverse drug reactions, or do we observe without treatment, with the chance of chronic ear disease and other complications? Do we immunize the child? There are lots of choices along the way, and you are not going to approve of all of them. The wellness-care mode of practice makes it clear to me that this patient is not my child, and his parents' choices are not my choices, but most of the time that's all right. When their choices aren't all right, we have to retain the old role and the old authority of the physician. This may entail being stern and directive with a family paralyzed by conflict or indecision. Once in a while it is necessary to report a family to a child abuse agency. When noncompliance becomes neglect, the counselor's role must give way, and the doctor becomes the child's advocate and an agent of the police power of the state.

What seems to work best for me is a melding of the old "Doctor Authority" and new "Doctor Facilitator." I don't find it necessary to outline the pros and cons of treating every case of impetigo or acute appendicitis, but I have gotten used to remaining open to discussing the options for handling "organic" problems. It is no longer so difficult to move into the facilitator mode when the issue is a sleep problem or obesity. So in this unexpected way, my experience with wellness care has informed and changed the way I function as a physician in general. Sometimes I miss the old Father-Knows-Best medicine, but in the long run a more democratic style seems to fit me and my families more comfortably. I commend it to you as well; you may like it.

❧ CHAPTER 7

Managing Well-Child Visits

In Chapter 3 I discussed at some length the time constraints in pediatric practice. Nowhere is this a bigger problem than in well-child care; there is no limit to the amount of time that can be spent on the problems of raising kids, but there is certainly a limit to the amount that anyone can afford. I assume that your well-child visits will last at least the 7 minutes that one study revealed to be the most common length of the pediatric-patient interaction; perhaps on occasion you will schedule 45 minutes or an hour for a complicated teenager. But no matter how much time you allow, the usual experience is that you could have used more; you will have to decide what you wish to accomplish during a well-child visit, and you will have to set priorities. Needless to say, the parent or the adolescent also has a priorities list, explicit and written down or unstated and hardly conscious.

How the visit is used should be the product of what all of you have in mind. The most important implication of this is entering the visit with an open ear, willing and ready to hear what the parent or the patient needs to say. I find this easiest to do by starting with an open-ended statement that invites response. Sometimes it is very general: "What's it like these days, now that he's crawling all over the house?" "Well, a whole year's gone by; how are you feeling about your first year as a parent?" Sometimes I'm more specific: "How are you managing to survive with the twins?" Sometimes I'll pick up an old thread: "How are things going with her night waking?" The trouble with that degree of specificity is that if she is still awakening five times a night and the parent feels like a guilty failure (and an incipient infanticidal maniac), it might have been better to address easier matters first. Perhaps the most important aspect of one's greeting question is the absolute necessity of avoiding the phrase "Do you have any problems?" Strange as this may sound, patients do not want to tell their doctors that they have problems. The very powerful impulse is to wish to appear healthy and happy, despite the competing desire to obtain information or relief of symptoms or a cure from the physician. It is as if we patients want to please our doctors by being successfully well. I vividly remember the first time I went for a general checkup to an internist friend clutching my little list of somatic complaints. It embarrassed me to have so many problems, so I omitted mention of the last three. So when you ask a young mother whether she has any problems, she will be likely to protect her image and her self-esteem by denying that there are any difficulties at all. She wants to feel good about herself as a mother, and she wants her pediatrician to validate her conduct; if she admits to having problems, how can she feel successful and competent?

A little list like the one that I carried to (and hid from) my doctor will often make an appearance in your office. Sometimes it will be so long that the items on *your* list, that is to say the issues you'd hoped to touch on during the visit, will never have a chance to surface. With each family, you learn how to balance your agenda with theirs. You also become aware that the most difficult questions may not be raised until the end of the session. Freud called these the "hand-on-the-doorknob" questions: "Oh, by the way, Doctor, Johnny seems to be awfully interested in lighting fires these days, and the local fire department asked me to mention this." It grieves me to admit this, but there is no good way to handle these terminal questions. If you say, "Sit down, Mrs. Plotz, and tell me more," you have just wiped out the rest of your morning schedule. If you say, "That sounds like something we need to talk about further; please tell the receptionist to set up a half-hour talk appointment this week," you may be perceived to be uninterested or unsympathetic. You also take the chance that the parent will decide not to pursue the matter. Take your choice of these unsatisfactory responses.

Fire-setting aside, there will be many issues to discuss that either you or the parents may wish to keep private from Johnny. This begins at a remarkably early age. The receptive vocabulary of a toddler is always much greater than anyone in the family imagines, and the discussion "over the child's head" of any sensitive topic must be considered to have been shared with the child. Any number of times, parents have reported behavior changes in 1- to 2-year-olds that certainly seemed to follow instantly from overheard adult talk. It is amusing to see how we adults respond to this problem. The use of a foreign language for private matters has been a standard stratagem in immigrant families; it works for a while. Sometimes I see parents lowering their voices and using a stage whisper, apparently hoping that the children will ignore them; it is a wonderful tribute to the power of wishful thinking. In the office, I try to handle the problem of privacy by sending the child out to the waiting room to play or to the nurse for tests or shots. This is by no means a satisfactory solution. The child under 3 years of age cannot be trusted to wander around the office unsupervised. Furthermore, many children aged 3 to 6 years resist being banished from the parent's presence because of either fear or the well-founded understanding that private matters concerning them will be discussed. Watching how parent and child handle this separation gives a nice insight about how limits are set and how coping behavior is elicited.

The well-child visit gives many other opportunities to observe family functioning. The interplay among children and parents reveals how power is distributed, how the parents treat each other, how decisions are made, and where the rough places exist in a marriage. When both parents and all the kids are present at the same time, a family's patterns of life become explicitly visible, sometimes painfully so.

Besides providing the practitioner with a crash course in family dynamics, the well-child visit gives the opportunity to monitor the important facets of the child's growth and development—physical, emotional, and mental. It is the vehicle for teaching the family about nutrition, safety, body care, preventive medicine, developmental patterns, sibling interaction, and whatever else strikes you as important for them to think about. From the family's point of view, it is, first and foremost, the time to find solutions to problems with the children. Some of these problems are of a straightforward "medical" nature: What makes his nose run all the time? What is this rash? Straightforward medical answers often suffice: He has sinusitis. The rash is impetigo. The problem is diagnosed and treatment can follow. However, many problems are found to involve family belief systems, parental disagreements, societal values, religious teachings, and intergenerational conflict, just to name a few of the possible factors: Should she be sleeping through the night? What about pacifiers? When should I wean him? Is it o.k. for Sarah and Sam to bathe together when they are 2 and 3 years old? How about at ages 5 and 6? Ages 8 and 9? These are not questions with unequivocal medical answers; they have to do with the way we choose to lead our lives.

If this is the case, it isn't the doctor's job to provide answers; it's our job to provide clarity. We can do this by pointing out the real issue. Recently, for example, a father wanted me to give him precise guidelines for the calorie and protein intake that his 9-year-old son should be allowed to have. It seemed like an unusual question until it became clear that the plump father was actually concerned with the possibility that his son would become overweight. This led to a discussion of the eating patterns of tall, skinny, active kids, like his, and the necessity of providing the right diet in an atmosphere of trust, rather than one of coercion and control. After defining the issue at hand, the next task is often to explore past efforts at reaching a solution. As every dermatologist knows, you don't make the mistake of prescribing the salve that has already failed. You also may need to discover whose views are involved in the definition of the problem. Does the question about toilet training come from the parent who is present, or does it come from the mother-in-law or the sitter? The answer may not satisfy everyone, but you need to know from which direction the wind is blowing, if only to give mom ammunition to use when she returns home to the query, "Well, what did the doctor say?"

When the problem has been defined, its history elucidated, and the various players identified, one can begin to discuss the various approaches to a solution. Two things are required: you must have some ideas about what might work, and you must understand that this is the family's problem, not yours. Sometimes a discussion about the options proceeds with the parent talking about his or her ideas, which you comment on in the light of your knowledge and experience: "No, serving the brussels sprouts cold the next day for breakfast isn't really likely to broaden his intake of cooked vegetables." Sometimes you will list the options yourself, with a clear statement about the pros and cons of each. This process makes it obvious that the family must decide how a problem is approached; it has to suit them, regardless of whether it would have suited you. It can be particularly difficult to remember this when the problem is too close to home for the doctor; the fact that my kid had the same problem should have nothing to do with what parents decide to do for their kids.

I've been implying that the problem-solving approach is a collaboration between a rational parent and a nondirective practitioner, but some parents are far from rational, and I know that I am rarely wholly nondirective. The parent's lack of rationality may be obvious, like that of the fat father, mentioned earlier, who had not noticed that his son was very slender. It can be harder to see, as in one mother who was having a terrible time setting limits for her toddler. She finally identified the problem as reflecting the brutal way in which her parents had disciplined her and her fear that she would be equally brutal if she set any rules at all. When reasonable approaches to ordinary family problems fail and fail and fail, you have to ask what is getting in the way. It may be unadmitted family conflict, parental neurosis or psychosis, drug use, conflicting cultural beliefs, or simple mental defect. It can also be an expression of family poverty or family disorganization.

About the practitioner's lack of absolutely nondirective objectivity, there is not much to say. I try to stay aware of my prejudices and label them when they surface, and I'm sure that my patients are aware of them as they get to know me. I take a little comfort from an old Southern pediatrician who told a colleague of mine, "When you see patients, tell them your opinion; that's what they pay you for."

Our objectivity or lack of it is one small part of the topic of our personal responses to a parent, a patient, or a family. In Chapter 4 on pediatrician-patient relationships, I mentioned the problem of families one dislikes. There are also families one likes too much. Sometimes this leads to so much identification that one begins to lose the necessary distance. I recall a talk appointment with parents, one of whom was a child psychiatrist, who had been my personal friends since college; they had come to discuss some problems with their daughter. Having briefly and uncomfortably heard their concerns, I offered soothing words, and my psychiatrist friend remonstrated, "Elmer, don't rush into premature reassurance!" He was absolutely correct.

The truth of the matter is that our personal, emotional responses to the people, adults or children, who we meet in our practices will be as varied as our responses to everyone else in our lives. How we manage the feelings evoked in us is a different issue; if we learn anything during medical training, it is that we must maintain a certain emotional distance and a kind of careful neutrality with patients. That is a true and valuable lesson; these people have sought us out not to find a new friend, a new lover, or a new enemy, but to obtain medical care. In the process of providing that care we will experience many emotional states, and some of them will not really belong to us. I am referring to a kind of emotional contagion that passes between patients and doctors. When you notice yourself becoming unexpectedly sad or angry or tense during a patient's visit, consider the possibility that you have picked up the emotional state of the other. If you are feeling particularly brave, you might try asking directly how the other person is feeling; the answer can be illuminating.

It may also take a certain bravery to talk to a patient with whom you are having a chronically unsatisfactory relationship. When I groan on noticing a particular patient's name on my daily schedule, it means that there are unresolved problems in my relationship with that child or, more often, those parents. It is also likely to mean that those parents or that child has some problems with me. On rare occasions I have had the good sense to broach the subject myself, instead of hoping that they would leave my practice. Even more rarely, this has led to a better relationship; there is absolutely nothing to lose by doing it.

One specific emotion worth mentioning is the sense of being burdened by a patient's problem. I know that some problems are painful, some terribly worrisome, some frighteningly challenging; those are all part of the package of practice. I am referring to a different feeling, which comes from being too closely identified with the child or his family; one feels as if one were carrying them on one's back. When you leave a visit with this heavy, laden, bent-back sensation, it is time to redefine the situation. You will need to distance yourself emotionally, enough to regain the neutrality that enables you to be a useful physician rather than a burnt-out acquaintance.

An old, sexist maxim of medicine is that it is hardest to provide care for famous people and beautiful women. (I imagine that heterosexual women doctors may have similar problems with beautiful men and that parallel problems exist for gay and lesbian physicians.) This is partly because people in these categories have different expectations of the world; they expect a certain amount of deference, a certain bending of the rules in their favor, a different power relationship with the rest of humankind. I find myself becoming uncomfortably aware of the physician-patient relationship when I see these folks; my usual absolute lack of self-consciousness flies away, and part of me watches the whole situation. It reminds me of the feelings I often had in training, those of observing the scene with a sense of, "Gee, I'm being a doctor." This makes for crummy care. Unfortunately, there does not seem to be any good solution to this dilemma. Eventually, one gets to know Mr. or Ms. Beautiful or Famous as a human being, and the relationship settles down a bit. Nevertheless, at least for me, these folks remain in their own category: fun to take care of, but not necessarily easy.

I have been talking as if the entire wellness-care visit were verbal and relational, but I have not forgotten the physical exam, about which I have a few observations that should probably be carved in stone. **Grossman's First Law of Physical Examination: Be flexible about what you examine.** It is necessary to decide what to examine and when. I have had a hard time discarding the notion that every patient contact requires a "complete physical exam." I know, we were all taught, "If you don't put your finger in it, you'll put your foot in it." I remember hearing about the great consultant pediatrician who said that the difference between himself and the doctors who sent him patients was that he did a fundoscopic exam and took the blood pressure. This is all quite true; a complete physical exam is a thing of beauty and a joy forever, and all that. However, it is not something you need to repeat endlessly; you will not learn anything new often enough to repay your effort. In short, this is an area in which one needs to think about cost-effectiveness. I hope you will not think I mean that you should look only into the ear that is reported to hurt. What I mean is that you should tailor your examination to the situation at hand. The risk is that you will not look widely enough to note the pharyngitis that explains the impetigo or the perianal cellulitis, or the swollen spleen that explains the malaise and fever. You have to use some judgment, but that's at least half the battle in medicine.

Grossman's Second Law of Physical Examination: Be flexible

about where you do the examination. One of the shiniest pearls a professor ever handed me was Dr. Helen Gofman's admonition to examine every newborn at the mother's bedside. Nearly every time, you will leave the mother relieved and happy. When there is something to be unhappy about, at least she will be knowledgeable instead of uninformed. After infancy, when the baby is becoming stranger-anxious, do the exam with the baby on the parent's lap; the frightened child can put up with a great deal more doctoring in that comforting place.

Grossman's Third Law of Physical Examination: Be flexible about how your examination proceeds. I was taught to start at the head and work on down to the toes, a reasonable rule for a neophyte who might forget some part or other in haste or confusion. When one is no longer a beginner, one can tailor an evaluation to the needs of the moment. For example, if you know the baby is going to be screaming at you within a minute or so, listen to his heart first when you still have a chance to hear something there. If the infant is just shy rather than furious, you may do best to start at the feet, a very non-threatening place; work your way up slowly, and keep the head for last. Try not to make eye contact; let the poor kid pretend you're not there. When you plan to measure the blood pressure and the child is tense, save it until the very end of the exam; she will have begun to relax, and her blood pressure will have dropped 10 points.

Grossman's Fourth Law of Physical Examination: Be rigid about completeness when it is indicated. Every new patient deserves a complete physical exam. A patient with an evolving problem may not need a complete exam at every visit, but you had best do it from time to time: something major may have changed. Decide when you will check reflexes, fundi, extraocular muscles, blood pressure, hearing, and vision; these exams may not be done at each wellness-care visit, but you will want them done often enough to provide a baseline and to pick up early pathologic change.

Well, there is your road map. In the next chapter we embark on the journey.

❧ CHAPTER 8

The Perinatal Period

Caring for the Normal Newborn and Family

One of my favorite notions is that the basic unit of human life is the family, rather than the individual. Nothing exemplifies this better than pregnancy and birth. So much of what happens to that fetus and baby is determined by the circumstances and the people around it that it is impossible to consider the newborn, except in family terms.

Everyone is involved; parents, siblings, grandparents—you name it, and this is true even in our era of weakened extended family ties. The needs, problems, abilities, and expectations of a whole crew of folks provide the setting for the perinatal period. Of course, the mother's experience of her pregnancy and the birth itself is crucial. It is hardly necessary to say that pregnancies vary from desired, healthy, and normal to tragically mistaken and pathologic. When you first see the product of this process you may be meeting a baby planned for, expected, and desired by healthy parents in comfortable circumstances with a supportive family and friends. Then again, you may not; I leave to your imagination and memories the list of possible alternatives. Clearly, the way a mother approaches her newborn depends on what has come before. Her fears, her health, her self-confidence, her ideas about the future of herself and her family—all affect how she will be able to function as a mother. The more you know about this penumbra of circumstance, the better you will be able to serve the baby and family.

The father also arrives at the perinatal period with a full load of emotional baggage. If this is his first child, he is likely to be full of doubts and fears: Will the baby be normal? Can we afford it? When will my wife go back to work? What kind of a father will I be? What kind of a kid will this infant turn into? Will my wife ever be interested in sex again? If there are other children and they have any imagination at all, they understand that life around the house will never be the same again. During their mother's pregnancy, they have probably gone through a number of changes. Sometimes, the older children have decided that a new baby is a pretty neat idea; sometimes, they watch their mother's swelling belly with apprehension and dismay. Marx said that no ruling class gives up power without a revolution, and this applies precisely to the situation in a one-child family that is becoming a two-child family. It is a big help if parents know this, and, as hard as this is to believe, some of them don't.

When a newborn is being adopted, a lot of emotional learning may have to be compressed into a brief period of time. When parents live through the biologic experience of the pregnancy, an emotional attachment to the baby develops as the fetus grows; this is perhaps especially true for the mother, but it happens to the father and the other children as well. Many times, adoption takes place precipitously, with arrangements being made within a few days before the infant's birth. This can make it more difficult for the family to become emotionally ready for the newcomer.

A nontraditional family will have nontraditional problems. The lesbian couples in our practice have to cope with new definitions of parenting; are they both "Mom" to the baby? The most important factor for these families may be the presence or absence of a supportive lesbian community.

The next facet to consider is where the birth will take place. I know that the vast majority of American babies will continue to be born in hospitals in the foreseeable future, and I don't doubt the wisdom of that practice for the safety of mothers and babies. However, I must say that home births have something to teach us. The preponderance of successful vaginal deliveries without the necessity of transferring the mother to a hospital for an operative delivery is the first consideration. Having one's labor in a familiar place, attended by a skilled midwife or physician, is clearly conducive to normal births. When I have come to see the new baby born at home, I have often been moved by the nearly palpable love and togetherness among the friends and family who are present. There is a primeval power involved in having one's baby at home; we lose that in our medicalized hospital births, and it is a real loss.

I recall coming into one bedroom when the baby was a few hours old; the mother was under the covers of the big bed, the two older children and the father all on top of the covers, the baby wrapped in a blanket, sleeping on the father's chest. It was like walking into the den of a tightly knit family of friendly bears. The children who are around the house during their mother's labor and birth have an instant attachment to the infant, which is wonderful to behold. Something similar can happen in a hospital's family-centered birth unit, but it takes some doing. The whole hospital atmosphere militates against the family. They are surrounded by machinery and by experts in uniforms; the ambience is cool and technical, one of applied science. The family members nearly inevitably feel superfluous, and often somewhat cowed. Structuring an environment that welcomes and supports the family means that we have to listen to their needs and perceptions, even when it conflicts with our usual ways of running obstetric and nursery services.

The other problem with hospital births is that, after having arranged to have the babies born there, we immediately throw them out. There was plenty wrong with the hospital routines of the past, but at least the mothers had a few days of rest, to be taken care of, and, with a little luck, to be given some useful instruction in the necessary arts of feeding and caring for infants. Early discharge certainly eliminates all that. The mother goes home exhausted, her milk not yet in and the baby just about to become jaundiced. It is unlikely that enough help is awaiting them. Predictably, the baby has a dreadful, fretful first night at home (most babies do), and by the fourth day post partum, the mother has more than sufficient reason to have a good case of "fourth-day blues." Don't be too surprised to find her in tears when you telephone. In fact, don't wait for the fourth day to call; your unsolicited call a day or two after discharge is excellent preventive medicine. You will pick up problems, either the baby's or the mother's, early enough to intervene usefully, and the family will be immensely relieved to know that they are not wholly abandoned by their medical advisors.

Meanwhile, back at the hospital, we have a new baby on our hands. If your hospitals are like the ones I work in, the newborn is subject to an immediately imposed routine composed of equal parts of good medical intentions, fears of legal liability, and ancient ritual. I first became aware of the last component when I had the opportunity to contrast the rules at the hospital where I first saw newborn care during medical school and the hospital, 400 miles away, where I served my internship. At the medical school, every newborn was placed prone with the head lower than the body for the first hours of life. It was explained to us that this allowed secretions to drain and avoided the risk of aspiration, which seemed reasonable enough to me. One year later, when I walked into the newborn nursery at the other hospital, the babies were supine, with their heads elevated. It was explained to me that this avoided the risk of aspiration. At that precise moment I began to understand why my medical school admissions interviewer had laughed when I told him I wanted to work in medicine, where science was applied to human needs.

In short, more than science is involved in our rituals. We skate on a thin ice of knowledge over a deep sea of ignorance. My point is that we should look critically at the interventions of the period immediately after birth. There is a lot to be said for leaving the parents and the baby alone; a healthy and unsedated infant is a remarkably sentient and responsive little creature, and her parents are exceedingly ready and eager to get to know her. After the briefest evaluation to ensure that cardiorespiratory function is adequate, a baby can be dried and wrapped a bit and given back to the mother. If one quietly observes the newly forming family relationships in these first minutes and hours, the special quality of the event becomes clear. It is a powerful time in which attachment is being established among mother, father, and baby (and siblings if they are present.) Among some medical people, there has been considerable resistance to this concept of "bonding." I think it has been hard for us to get out of the way, give up our necessary but intrusive medical roles, and leave the new family alone. Perhaps it is also the case that obstetricians and delivery room nurses can become desensitized to the excitement and specialness of birth. After the first few hundred deliveries, babies and mothers may look pretty much alike to a tired practitioner at 2:00 in the morning; the family's alleged need for quiet time together may seem unimportant.

Among the medical rituals of the newborn period, a complete physical exam done as soon as possible during the first day of life certainly makes sense. This is true not only from a medical point of view but also because the parents nearly always have questions about their new baby, and usually a certain amount of anxiety as well. "Is everything normal?" is the unspoken question in the parents' minds. For this reason, the first exam should be done with the infant on the mother's bed. During the exam, I tell the parents what I'm looking at or listening to, and I tell them my findings as I proceed. Most of the time, this is a wonderfully reassuring experience for the parents. If you don't do the exam in their presence, it is difficult for some mothers to believe that their babies are really all right. Of course, sometimes everything isn't all right. The discovery of an anomaly during a bed-side exam does put the doctor on the spot; one lacks the time for a considered statement or for consultation with a handy textbook. This is a disadvantage that seems to me worth accepting. During your examination of the baby, observe the parents as well: How are they responding? Does the mother reach out spontaneously to touch her baby? What comments do they make? This is an emotionally charged event: don't expect either parent to retain any specific information from you. If what you tell them needs to be remembered, write it down.

Actually, writing your instructions and other information is a necessity during every hospital visit with the mother and baby. The mothers in most American hospitals are the recipients of endless advice from everyone around them. You may even agree with some of the advice, but don't count on it. What the lady who visits the mother in the adjoining bed tells your patient is probably as memorable as what you tell her. Give your advice an edge: leave a printed or written copy for the family to peruse and take home. I like to use a printed outline on which I make notes appropriate to the particular family. It is included in the back of this book, Appendix A.

The first topic is food. If the mother is nursing, there is much to be said, and the next chapter covers this subject. If the baby is formula-fed, the choice of formula is likely to be a "humanized" cow's milk, like Similac, Enfamil, or SMA. Only iron-containing preparations should be used; nobody needs anemia. If there is allergy in parents or other close relatives, it probably makes sense to use soy-based formula or casein hydrolysate (Nutramigen), although the expense of the latter is painful. The preparations easiest to use are the concentrates, mixed half and half with warm tap water in an unsterile but clean bottle, and made for one feeding at a time when needed. If the concentrate is kept refrigerated after opening until use, the water supply is safe, and the bottle is consumed within about 2 hours after mixing, there is no need for anything to be sterilized. Preparing an unsterile bottle with warm tap water takes about 1 minute, if one works leisurely. The absence of a sterilization ritual will distress a number of grandmothers, but it has no other disadvantage. If the local water supply is fluoridated, make sure that the family knows this and uses it; the only kids in my practice with severe caries were raised on purchased bottled water. If you don't have fluoridation, prescribe a fluoride supplement and, as often as you can, remind the family to use it; people forget the little bottles. (Alternatively, organize a community campaign for fluoridation; fluoride supplements aren't going to reach many of the children that fluoridated water would have protected.)

What goes in must come out. Don't forget to tell parents what to expect about the newborn's stools. I usually mention that some babies produce their stools with accompanying groans and grunts that signify nothing.

Another topic is household environment. Babies thrive in houses from Louisiana in August to Nome in January. The rule is to dress them to fit the circumstances, and they will adapt. They do not need the hothouse steam bath that some cautious parents provide.

Why bathe a baby every day? Americans worry too much about germs and dirt. Most infants do very well with a bath every few days, although an occasional baby gets a scruffy case of seborrhea unless a daily bath is given. There is no need for fancy and expensive soaps; any mild soap is fine. "Baby" shampoos are buffered to avoid conjunctival irritation; it makes sense to use them to wash the infant's head and face. One sacroscant piece of nonsensical ritual advice is to avoid a tub bath until the navel has healed. There is something about navel magic that breeds belief in ritual rules; why, for example, should the diaper be folded to avoid touching the remnant of cord? and why should a ritual anointment of rubbing alcohol be placed on or about the poor shriveled little thing? Navels have healed in every mammalian species for some years now without our well-meaning advice. This may be stated in a more general way as **Grossman's First Law of Medicine: Resist the urge to medicalize normal processes.**

The remaining topics I want to touch on are family rather than infant matters. Families need to know that peace and quiet are precious and that every one of their friends and family will want to come to see the new baby immediately, thereby making peace and quiet impossible to attain. The needs conflict; parents and the new baby need settling-down time to get to know each other, to allow the natural rhythms to become established, and to let the tired mother rest. All true, but the need to view the newborn is amazingly powerful: "We'll just drop by for a few minutes" is well-intentioned but dishonest. A partial solution is to schedule a visiting day a week or so later, but people generally find this hard to do. One mother (who had been raised in the military) posted a notice on her front door advising any visitors that "by order of her pediatrician" no visitors would be allowed for the first fortnight. It was an impressive document but was unrepresentative of parents as a group. New mothers need to be told to nap whenever they have the chance; thank-you notes can wait. They also need to know that this is the time to get all the household help possible, so that they can concentrate on their own recovery and the needs of the baby.

The last thing I tell the new parents is that I'll be telephoning them in a day or so and making a house call a few days thereafter. Knowing that they are not completely alone with the newborn is remarkably comforting to inexperienced and shaky parents.

The timing of the follow-up telephone call depends on the baby's condition, the family's level of anxiety, and how busy I happen to be. This last criterion sounds crass and unprofessional, which it is. It is also realistic. The middle of the winter influenza epidemic has a number of demands that may have to come first. However, a telephone call a day or two after the baby goes home is welcome and timely. I want to know about feeding pattern, stools, urine, appearance of jaundice, and general infant behavior. The parent's answers give me a good idea of how they are holding up. During the telephone call, I'll usually decide when to make a house call. No, that is not a misprint; we do make new-baby house calls, to the utter amazement of families new to our practice. Like other primary care physicians, we used to make house calls routinely, on sick kids as well as neonates. Like everybody else, we pretty much abandoned illness house calls decades ago.

Newborn house calls are a different matter, and we doggedly hang on to this excellent tradition. This is largely because we learn so much about the families we visit; the family in situ is very different from the family in the doctor's office. How you live is who you are, and no matter how frantically you clean up the living room in anticipation of the doctor's visit, you can't really hide the realities of your life. Sometimes the previously hidden reality is financial; I recall a few home visits in which the home turned out to be a mansion and a few in which the depth of poverty revealed was nearly unbelievable. Sometimes I was greeted by the chaos of severe mental illness. I will never forget the house full of garbage—on the floor, all over the kitchen, in the fireplace—and the unkempt child lying on a couch under a carefully drawn picture of an infant reaching for a black widow spider. The house call on the newborn provides the opportunity to see how everyone in the family is functioning: parents, baby, siblings, and the family dog. If you make your visit during the first week, you will find a substantial incidence of "fourth-day blues," and your support may be critically helpful when everything is beginning to fall apart. You will also discover nursing problems that would have defeated the mother if left untreated until your routine office visit in a few weeks. Sometimes, you will find a sick infant whose undemanding behavior had been considered that of a "good baby."

I take an interval history, and I do a complete physical exam with the entire family in attendance. Afterward, I'll reinforce any previously given advice that seems to be needed and remind the parents to set up the well-baby appointments. If there are problems, I make a note to call back to check on their solutions. In part because house calls are so unexpected and unusual, the whole event is a ritual that brings us all closer together. It means a great deal to the family; parents talk about the newborn house call for years and years. If there are older siblings, the house call is important for them as well. Children love seeing their doctors in their own homes; we clearly seem much safer and less threatening to them on their own turf. Bring some little presents for them. In my house call bag I carry some of the prizes kids in our office receive when they get shots: stickers, plastic animals, little rings. During a time when everyone is making a great fuss over the new baby, the older kids appreciate a little symbolic attention, too.

❧ CHAPTER 9

Helping Mothers Nurse Their Babies

It strikes me as odd that there is any necessity for a chapter about helping mothers to nurse. I suppose it is the result of two social trends; first, the popularization of formula-feeding, which resulted in a couple of generations of grandmothers who could not teach their daughters what they themselves did not know; second, the sexualization of the breast, which has become so complete that young women have to relearn and newly experience their bodies as being nurturing as well as sexual. The first of these factors is a perfect example of the hazards of medicalizing life, turning the most basic female function into an infrequently chosen and ill-understood alternative to a factory-produced, medically supervised, and highly advertised commercial product. The second factor has its effect on the male physician, who probably shares the general American view that the breast is mostly an object to be shared by consenting adults and hardly the proper place for babies. Somehow, we male physicians have to graduate to a more neutral position, just as we do about the female body in general.

Most of the pregnant women I meet at prenatal visits have already made up their minds about nursing. Many are wondering whether they can combine nursing with formula-feeding, so that they can return to work or so that the baby's father can share the feeding. It is necessary to be realistic about these plans. A highly demanding, full-time job away from home makes it difficult for a mother to keep her milk supply going. Even if she can express milk a few times during the workday and bring it back to the baby, the physical demands of her life as mother and worker may be excessive. The idea of sharing

51

feeding with father tends to work in the latter part of the first year when the baby is close to sleeping through the night; in the early months, most mothers have so much milk production during the night that they want to nurse, just for their own comfort.

The other uncertainties one hears are "Can I really nurse the baby?" and "Do I really want to?" These are large and complex questions that may stem simply from lack of experience with other mothers' successful nursing; for the woman who was herself bottle-fed and whose peers have chosen to bottle-feed, the lack of role models is daunting. The questions may also have psychological meanings not easily accessible to the woman herself. I have learned to proceed cautiously in these situations; I don't know why she doesn't want to nurse, and I don't want to push her into a decision that may not make sense to her. Nursing undertaken because of family or medical pressure is likely to fail, and everyone ends up defeated. Perhaps the wisest course is to try to clarify the options for the family and recommend other sources of information. The innumerable books on breast-feeding are useful, as is help from the nursing mothers' group, La Leche League. Advocates of nursing, like advocates of whales and handguns, can tend to be a bit zealous, and I like to warn the parents to take the advice they get with some caution.

In the last months of pregnancy, nipple and breast preparation is helpful. Breasts that have always been protected from wind and weather are ill-prepared to withstand the attack of a hungry newborn. Scrubbing the nipples during a shower or vigorously toweling them afterward can reduce sensitivity. Carefully limited sun exposure may also be useful. In the weeks just before term, expressing colostrum appears to facilitate the beginning of nursing. I warn the mothers to stop if uterine contractions are noted.

After the baby is born, early and frequent nursings help to bring the milk in quickly and may minimize breast engorgement. The baby's rooming-in as much as possible during the hospital stay makes it easier to nurse on demand. The length of time on the breast depends on the mother's skin color. The white-skinned strawberry-blond will have very sensitive nipples and should nurse only a few minutes at each breast at first; the darker the skin color, the less sensitive the nipples. Nursing times will increase as the baby wakes up and gets hungrier and as the mother tolerates longer feeds. Eventually, most

American babies nurse 5 to 20 minutes at each breast 6 to 12 times a day; it may take days or weeks for an infant to have the stamina to take both breasts at a feeding. Our expectations of infant feeding have been skewed by the decades of experience with artificially fed babies. The bottle-fed infant works much less hard to get a meal, and the big feeding of slowly digested formula stays longer in the stomach. For these infants, five to seven feeds a day are often sufficient, and a schedule of 3- to 5-hour feedings develops. In contrast, the small meals of rapidly digested, low-protein breast milk are required much more often. In primitive societies in which the baby is nearly always next to the mother, feedings of 20 or more times a day are standard. Giving bottles of anything to normal, full-term newborns is deleterious to nursing. Contrary to nursery mythology, one cannot prevent physiologic jaundice with water or glucose supplements. The only indication for p.c. liquids is nipple soreness so severe that nursing time must be limited.

This brings us to the uncomfortable subject of sore nipples. During the first days of nursing, most mothers experience some nipple pain, especially at the start of a feeding as the baby gets the nipple firmly in its mouth. Holding the infant so that the entire nipple can be in the baby's mouth is a help; the baby who chews on the end of the nipple is an inefficient and painful nurser. This situation can be avoided by holding the baby's body a little above the breast with the mother's arm well-supported by pillows. This allows the baby's head and mouth to fall into the breast. It is practically never necessary to hold the breast away from the baby's nose; they manage to breath nicely even when surrounded by the most pillowly bosoms.

Normal nipple sensitivity can be helped a bit by heat; a hair blow-dryer, a bright lamp, or a little sunlight all can be soothing. Exposure to air is also helpful. Nipple shields should be avoided if at all possible; once used, they are very hard to get rid of, because the baby learns to depend on them. The new, very thin models are least objectionable, because they allow more normal nursing. A wonderful variety of creams and liquids have been proposed for local application to sore nipples; none does much good for the usual case, and some are actively harmful. Hydrous lanolin is benign, but not much more. The best advice is to minimize washing, especially with soap, and forget about nipple creams, unless the nipples become excessively red, sore, and cracked. In those instances, an ointment containing an anti-inflammatory steroid and an antiyeast antibiotic can be rapidly helpful. This should be applied sparingly after each nursing, and not washed off. Very rarely there will be a component of bacterial infection, for which one can add an antibacterial ointment. If the mother develops signs of a possible breast abscess, medical assistance will be needed for diagnosis and treatment.

Most important here is that the mother know where to turn for help. This is largely a question of local protocol, I suppose. My rule is to treat nipple problems, because they come to my attention as part of the management of nursing, but I ask the mother to call her obstetrician or family doctor about a possible breast infection that might require a systemic antibiotic for her. During the 1950s and 1960s when nursery infections with virulent staphylococci were common, maternal breast infections became a major problem. This now is a relatively rare occurrence, and treatment with an antistaph antibiotic is curative. We learned in that previous era that mothers could and should continue to nurse during the infection; the milk from the affected breast does no harm to the baby, and the infection clears more rapidly when the breast is emptied by the baby. A plugged milk duct will cause the development of a tender, hard, and sometimes reddened area at the periphery of the breast. This mimics the beginning of a breast abscess, but the absence of fever, chills, and malaise suggests that the problem is just mechanical plugging rather than infection. The mother should massage the blocked segment of the breast while nursing, pressing gently toward the nipple. Hot compresses applied as few times a day help to relieve pain.

A major component of nursing comfort is the mother's posture and support. If she is physically tense during nursing and if she supports the baby's weight without assistance, nursing will be a tiring process. However, if the mother can find a comfortable chair with arms that, suitably pillowed, can do the job of propping the baby in place, the nursing period can be one of physical rest and relaxation. Watch the posture she assumes; the mother's arms and shoulders should look and feel relaxed. I tell mothers that nursing should be a one-armed procedure, leaving her other hand free to hold a book, the telephone, or a glass of beer. The reference to the beer is deliberate (more about it later); many mothers report intense thirst accompanying the act of nursing, especially during the first weeks. Mothers sometimes report a shiver or a chill when their milk lets down; this is harmless and disappears with time. The last point about nursing technique is to keep clothes and bedding out of the way during the first days of nursing. The baby needs to feel and smell the breast, and this can be pretty hard to manage if brassiere, sheets, blankets, and nightgowns keep falling over his nose.

Mothers often are concerned about the quality and quantity of their milk. Quality is a nonissue; breast milk is not a uniform product, but it is always adequate in quality for a term infant. Quantity is another matter. Certainly the vast majority of women can and do produce enough milk in the early post-term period, but there really are a few women who are not good nursers. Some of them have nipples so flat or inverted that the baby cannot nurse effectively; some just don't make much milk. This should not come as a surprise; even mammals bred for milk production vary in ability to make milk.

A decrease in milk production should be suspected when a mother who has been nursing successfully for weeks or months reports that the baby is fretful at the breast—especially in the afternoon or evening, that the baby's stools and urine are diminishing, or that nursing frequency has increased and the baby is again awakening at night to feed. The usual factors leading to a decrease in breast milk are maternal exhaustion, inadequate maternal diet, and infrequent nursing. Sometimes special circumstances inhibit milk production, such a mother-in-law's visit or other psychological stresses. Depending on the particular causes, some or all of the following advice may be given:

1. Increase maternal rest time; get an afternoon nap, if possible.

2. Hire or beg some help; get someone to do the shopping, cooking, and cleaning for a while. This may be a relative, a husband, a friend, or a local high school student.

3. Eat! Mothers need three meals a day. Fluids, as such, do not need to be stressed; one's natural thirst will ensure fluid intake. Calcium intake is important in the long run for maternal health, but it does not seem to matter for milk pro-

duction. Mothers are often under considerable pressure to lose weight in the early postnatal period; a calorie-restricted diet will predictably diminish breast milk.

4. Brewer's yeast is a time-honored folk remedy that works. Take one tablet t.i.d. at first, and slowly increase to three tablets t.i.d., if tolerated. Too much yeast causes cramps and flatus in some women.

5. Beer is a specific galactogogue that has been shown[1,2] to increase prolactin production; drink 6 to 12 ounces one or two times a day. The alcohol in beer may sedate the baby so it is best not to drink it just before nursing. De-alcoholized beer may be used, if desired.

6. Other medications, most recently metoclopramide, have been proposed as galactogogues, but I have not found them useful.

7. Oxytocin nasal spray can be used if the mother has difficulty in letting her milk down; this is an uncommon problem.

8. Increase the frequency of nursings: the more feedings per day, the greater the milk volume will be. Even brief feedings are helpful.

9. Give the baby as little supplemental formula as you can.

10. Get rid of unwanted mothers-in-law, if possible.

It takes about 2 to 3 days to begin to obtain a satisfactory return of adequate breast milk. It is not usually necessary to continue all these measures indefinitely, but recurrent episodes of decreased milk may be expected.

One strange instance of nursing failure is the baby who starves at the breast. These infants somehow fail to indicate to their mothers that they are grossly undernourished. Sometimes the mother clearly does not want to see what is happening. This is a dangerous and

[1] De Rosa G et al: Prolactin Secretion After Beer. Lancet 1981;ii:934.
[2] Carlson HE et al: Beer-Induced Prolactin Secretion. J Clin Endocrinol Metab 1985;60:673–677.

delicate situation; one needs to protect the infant, but one does not want to upset the mother. Keep in mind that a depressed or psychotic mother may be unable to act rationally in her baby's interests. Sometimes the mother is perfectly able to respond to the baby's needs, but the baby is too quiet and apathetic to get her attention. Monthly well-child visits with accurate weighings will alert you to these babies. Watch the growth charts carefully; the baby who is gaining relatively less weight than length is probably underfed. Parenthetically, the best growth charts provide an entire 8″ by 11″ page for the first year of life. We use the old University of Iowa charts from 1942, even though kids are a bit bigger these days.

At the other end of the spectrum is the mother who makes too much milk. This usually evens out within a few weeks as the breast supply diminishes to equal demand, but on occasion a baby is so over-fed that it will spit up impressive amounts after feedings. I once hospitalized an infant for suspected pyloric stenosis, whose only problem was surfeit. The solution in these circumstances is nursing only one breast at a feeding.

The mother of twins has innumerable special problems, among which nursing techniques are rather minor. Most mothers choose to nurse one baby at a time, either one breast per infant plus a supplementary bottle, if needed, or a bilateral nursing for one feeding alternating with a bottle at the next. Some mothers are adept at nursing both babies at once, but this takes some agility. The best advice you can give these families is to get in touch with other families with twins; the shared practical experience is invaluable, and maybe someone will lend them a double stroller.

Nursing premature babies who weigh about 4 pounds or more poses no particular difficulty. The smaller babies generally need to be started on gavage feedings or bottle feedings with "premie" nipples, with a gradual transition to the breast as the babies gain size and vigor. For very-small-birth-weight premies, there is some evidence that breast milk supplemented by the more concentrated premature formulas is superior to breast milk alone.

The mother who needs to express her milk may find manual expression tedious and difficult. A number of breast pumps are available, among which the stationary electric pumps are clearly most efficient; the little battery-operated pumps are not much good. Some models use alternating pressure and suction; this seems to be the most comfortable and fastest type. The manual devices use suction only and tend to be quite slow. The local chapter of La Leche League will be a good source of information on breast pump rentals or purchase.

A frequent problem is the safety of maternal medication. I must say that I don't worry much about this. Many medicines are excreted into the breast milk, usually in small amounts, but if it is something that one can safely give an infant, it does not seem worthwhile to interrupt nursing. Some drugs have noticeable but unimportant effects; maternal cathartics may loosen a baby's stool, and codeine may be mildly sedating. Obviously, mothers should not nurse when they are taking medications with a significant risk of toxicity to the baby; this would include antimetabolites, radioactive substances, tetracyclines, and some psychoactive agents. I think one has to balance risks. A depressed mother taking an antidepressant might be so distressed at having to stop nursing that a wiser choice would be to let her continue. Oral contraceptives pose a special problem: if taken during the first few months after childbirth, they often strongly inhibit milk production. The later in the first year they are started, the less this effect is noted.

Breast milk jaundice is an ill-understood entity to which too much attention is paid. When physiologic jaundice fails to subside in a breast-fed infant by the end of the first week or two of life, breast milk jaundice is certainly a likely cause. If there is no blood incompatibility and the baby is otherwise thriving, I often limit my search for alternative causes to a thorough physical exam plus a urinalysis and urine culture. Then one can take the baby off breast milk for 48 hours and monitor the bilirubin; it should drop promptly. The mother should then resume nursing; the bilirubin will increase, although rarely to the previously attained levels. As long as the indirect bilirubin remains below 20 mg%, there is no need for further intervention. Within a few weeks, perhaps 2 months at most, the baby's jaundice will be gone. If everyone is nervous about the persistent jaundice, one can give the baby phenobarbital, an excellent enzyme inducer; this will speed resolution of the problem.

Mothers whose babies are exclusively or largely breast-fed will not usually experience the resumption of menses for several months. When their first periods begin, some mothers report that the baby seems unhappy with nursing for a day or two; this is not related to any apparent change in milk volume, but presumably there is a change in smell or taste. The phenomenon is transient and usually does not recur with the succeeding menstrual periods.

A common problem in the middle of the first year of nursing is distractibility. An active and responsive baby may be so interested in the environment that he pulls away from the nipple every time the dog walks into the room or the telephone rings. Even worse, some babies turn away from the breast without letting go of the nipple. For these infants, nursing may need to be accomplished in a quiet and darkened room. However, this tends to be the baby who at an early age decides that nursing is too confining, and weans himself to the bottle.

The final issue is how long to nurse. This is a wonderfully complex issue. I remember our first child's pediatrician telling us that babies should be weaned from breast or bottle early in the second year "to avoid oral dependency." We were impressed at the time but soon recovered our skepticism when we realized that the data to support this rule were probably nonexistent. Weaning age is basically socially determined. Traditional Sioux Indians weaned their children at age 5 or 6 years. A New Guinea tribe with a prohibition against sexual intercourse during the months when the mother is nursing tends to wean by the middle of the first year, at the latest. It should be easy to sell them bottled formula. In short, every group has its own rules.

The baby also has something to say about this. Some infants really love to nurse and will give up the breast only with coercion. Others, especially very active babies, lose interest in nursing and wean themselves sometime in the first year. Fathers play a role as well. The nursing mother and her baby form a close bond that may exclude the father. He may also feel considerable sexual jealousy, especially since it can take so long for many new mothers to regain any interest in sex.

The mother's feelings about duration of nursing should be the defining factor. Every mother's experience of nursing is different. Some women love the whole process; they enjoy the physical sensations of the baby at the breast, and they feel fulfilled as women in a powerful way. For such a woman, giving up nursing is a real loss.

One mother of four children sat in my office and wept as she related that her 7-month-old son had abruptly weaned himself. "He is the last baby I'll ever nurse; now that I've gotten really good at being the mother of an infant, I'll never do it again and it seems such a waste." For other mothers, nursing is fine for feeding babies but means much less to them; it's easy to stop. For a few women, nursing is a chore that they undertake dutifully but without joy; they tend to wean early. Nursing can also be perceived as a considerable physical strain; only after weaning do some mothers regain their prepregnancy energy.

The process of weaning is straightforward. If the baby is older than about 12 to 18 months, it may be possible to wean to the cup. These days, most American babies are weaned to the bottle or a combination of bottle plus cup. A gradual replacement of breast milk with cow's milk is usually the easiest choice for everyone; a rapid change is likely to cause constipation, sore breasts, and hard feelings. The mother can substitute a bottle or cup for the least important nursing, and every week or so drop another nursing. Often the nursing that feels most important to mother or baby is retained for additional weeks. If the weaning process goes on for months, someone involved may need assistance in letting go. If it is the child, the parents may need your help in feeling free to give their baby a boost over a developmental hurdle. This is a paradigm for many such episodes in the child's life; some tasks look very difficult, and the parents' calm assurance that the child can master change and growth can be a big help. If the mother is holding on to nursing, it may be worthwhile to help her explore her reasons. The simple act of expressing her feelings in words may be enough to clarify her choices and let her make the change.

❧ CHAPTER 10

Well-Baby and Well-Child Care

Like most American pediatricians in largely middle class communities, I spend about half of my practice time providing "wellness care," the supervision, through regularly scheduled visits, of the growth and development of babies, children, and adolescents. This investment of time and money allows me to watch for and intervene against physical, behavioral, and emotional problems early in their genesis. It ensures that routine immunizations are done, if the parents haven't been frightened by a variety of quacks. I can measure growth, hearing, and vision, and check blood and urine for abnormalities. The frequent wellness-care visits provide a basis of knowledge and trust between the families and the pediatrician; after a short time, the parents learn that they have a reliable and often useful source of information about their child, and the doctor learns a great deal about the strengths and problems in each family in the practice. In time, the child also learns to trust and use the doctor; I always ask middle-aged and older children what questions they have about their growth and their health, and their responses become more and more sophisticated as they grow up.

Needless to say, wellness care is a great luxury. In most parts of the world, medical care is necessarily limited to serious illness: issues of normal growth and development or questions of family functioning have low priority when basic human needs are largely unmet. I must confess that I often have felt guilty to be spending so much energy and effort in this area of my medical life; I'm not saving lives when I'm seeing well babies. What I am doing is filling a need for medical and emotional support in a fragmented society in which weakened family structure and accelerating social change leave parents vulnerable and confused. I don't like "medicalizing" these normal aspects of human existence, but the absence of a stable and respected extended family or an agreed-upon set of cultural norms may make my answers the best support a family can obtain.

In the 12 sections that follow, I indicate the areas of interest to parents, children, and doctors at each stage of life from the newborn period to mature adolescence. I do not mean to imply that every subject can or should be raised at every well-child visit; on the contrary, we have to limit the scope of a visit to the time available and to the interests of the parent or the child. If you want to talk to the mother about home safety at the 8-month-old's visit and she wants to talk about the impending divorce, you had better put off your excellent advice regarding gates on the stairways. It is also necessary to limit the physical exam. A complete first physical exam for a new patient, whether a newborn or an older child, is an obvious responsibility and one of the reasons to insist on a long, comprehensive visit for each new patient. However, it is a waste of time to repeat a full exam every month during the first year. Ask yourself what may change, and focus your efforts there.

In the absence of symptoms, I look at skin, ears (lots of surprises there, even without symptoms), nose, mouth, teeth and throat, cervical nodes, heart and lungs (briefly), and abdomen and genitals; I glance at the extremities and back. On my first complete exam I look closely at head size and shape, and I depend on my memory to alert me to a change in the future. Extraocular motion should be looked at repeatedly during the first years, afterward only rarely if vision is normal. I do a fundoscopic exam at the first visit with a child over 3 years of age; before that I'll be satisfied with a brief peek, unless I have questions about vision or a serious abnormality. After the first complete look, a repeat fundoscopic exam every few years seems enough. My approach is similar for blood pressures; if the pulses and the heart seem normal, I get my first blood pressure reading at about age 1 year, and then every 5 years until adolescence, when I begin to take a reading every year. During the first year of life I check the foot reflexes frequently, because I'm interested in the relation of the plantar grasp and Babinski reflexes to standing and walking. Thereafter, I check muscle reflexes no more often than every few years. Backs can change: I check for scoliosis at least once a year, and I try to stay aware of back contour, even when I'm listening to a chest.

Regular measurements of weight are invaluable; unfortunately, this requires an accurate scale and a careful person doing the weighing. Many mistakes are made, and you will often have to re-weigh a child who has allegedly become lighter. The determination of length is even more error-prone. I ask our office nurses to measure well babies only every other month, because so often they are reported to have shrunk when monthly measurements are attempted. It is possible, but difficult and expensive, to measure vision and hearing in very small infants. Practically speaking, age 3 is about the earliest you can make the attempt. We use a little transistorized audiometer for hearing tests, and our nurses get good results by age 4, at the latest. Initial distant vision tests are done with standardized pictures at the same age. A fuller test of near and far vision, fusion, and eye coordination is done with a testing machine at age 4 or 5. If there is any reason to test color vision, that is best accomplished with Ishihara color cards at age 5 or older.

❧ EARLY INFANCY

Feeding

Breast-feeding is discussed in Chapter 9. Bottle-feeding in the United States today is usually a straightforward matter of giving a "humanized" cow's milk formula. Enfamil, Similac, and SMA are the commonly used brands; all of these should be used in the added iron formulation, unless you have convincing proof that the low iron formula is better-tolerated. In the presence of major allergy in either parent or with a considerable history of allergies in close family members, it is probably wise to avoid cow's milk-based formulas and cow's milk-based foods for the first year. Soy milks based on soy protein isolate like Isomil, I-Soyalac, and Prosobee are generally well-tolerated. Nutramigen, made from casein hydrolysate, is even less likely to induce an allergic response, but it is painfully expensive.

In early infancy, both parents and pediatricians tend to blame every symptom on a feeding problem. Sometimes this is indeed the case; vomiting, diarrhea, bloody stools, constipation, colic, eczema, and general unclassified misery are all possible complications of formula-feeding. However, the gastrointestinal tract is the final common pathway for the expression of other ills as well. Infection outside the gut, especially pyelonephritis, cardiovascular disease, and various metabolic abnormalities, come first to mind. Therefore, we need to think further than formula manipulation when a baby does not seem to tolerate formula feedings.

Some formula problems are truly allergy-related; any of the gastrointestinal symptoms already mentioned may occur, or typical infant eczema may develop with red, itchy cheeks and antecubital spaces or patchy dry nummular spots all over the body. At times you may be confused by a widespread case of seborrhea. The rash is usually a yellow, "crushed potato chip" scale with cradle cap, retroauricular scale and redness, pale or pink skin creases, and no itching. Unhappily, intermediate or mixed cases occur that are quite puzzling. I hedge my diagnosis, note "seborrheic eczema" in the chart, treat for seborrhea with frequent washing and possibly sulfur and salicylic acid shampoo, and await developments. If it is really allergic eczema, it will get worse. If the rash is eczema, switch the formula to soy or Nutramigen. Soy usually works, and it is usually well-tolerated, except for a tendency to cause green stools, but some milk-allergic babies are also allergic to soy, or they rapidly develop a soy allergy. Nutramigen is more likely to succeed, but the cost is burdensome for most families. If the symptoms are cured by one of these formula changes, you have good reason to suspect that this baby is an allergy-prone person. A prudent course is to delay the introduction of all solid foods until at least 5 months and preferably later, and to delay the use of the highly allergenic foods (wheat, egg, fish, shellfish, orange, peanut, all milk products, corn, chocolate) until as late as possible in the first year or later.

Constipation is only rarely a symptom of allergy, but it is probably the most common nonallergy-related problem with formula-feeding. The solution is generally simple: add extra carbohydrate to the feeding. This can be plain white sugar, about ½ to 1 teaspoon per bottle. If that fails, molasses at the same dose is usually effective; sometimes only one or two bottles a day will need to be laced with the molasses. Malt extract is also useful, but the volume required is much larger and the cost is high.

Behavior and Development

Aside from feeding, the areas of most interest to the parents of the new baby are behavior and development. As a pediatrician, I share their focus on the signs of normal function revealed by the baby's ability to fix gaze, track, respond to voices and other sounds, smile, and vocalize. The pace of acquisition of these and subsequent milestones of nervous system development tells us a great deal about the child. Perhaps equally important are the behavioral signs hinting at what sort of temperament the baby comes equipped with. I don't see much predictive value in the way a newborn acts; the exigencies of birth seem to be most important in shaping behavior during the first week or so; but within a very few weeks of life one can begin to make some fairly accurate guesses about a baby's personal style. This notion may seem odd to readers who were taught, as I was, that personality is largely shaped in family relationships. As a good Freudian, I had expected to understand children in terms of how they were raised by their parents. It came as a distinct surprise to me to observe that the crucial factors often seemed to be the inborn temperament of the child and how the family dealt with that already-defined reality. It was a further revelation to watch children over the years and to see how consistent their personalities remained. I learned this, in part, from the clinical studies of my late partner Percy Jennings. He recorded parents' and his own office observations of infant and early childhood behavior and correlated these data with parents' and psychologists' observations in later childhood and adolescence. Like Escalona at Menninger's and Thomas, Burch, and Chess in New York, he found impressive consistency over time.

I see the importance of this observation in two ways. First, it can help a family to become aware of the specific personality pattern of each child. The sooner you know what you have, the easier it may be to tailor your expectations and your style as the child's parent. If your first-born happens to be a peaceful, slow-moving, phlegmatic person with a long attention span, you may expect the next baby to follow a similar pattern. What if the second is an intrusive, active, socially hyper-responsive, generally high-pitched little dynamo? It becomes necessary to reframe expectations, lock up the poisons, get lots of baby gates, and generally change the way the household functions. The family that attempts to treat every child alike and expects every child to meet similar standards will have an unnecessarily hard time of child-rearing. I try to perceive the underlying patterns revealed by parental report and by what I can see in the office, and I show the parents what they may have been too close to see themselves.

The second way in which this point of view is important is in helping the parents to re-examine the notion that "I am totally responsible for everything good or bad in my child's life." This seems to me neither useful nor true. In American medicine during the recent phase of simple-minded, blame-the-parent theorizing about children's problems, we did a great deal of harm by telling the mothers of autistic kids that the autism was their fault, and we did similar harm to parents of children with anorexia or migraine or peptic ulcer. A closer approximation of truth may be that particular children have particular tendencies and that the best we parents can do is help them to cope with who they are.

Colic

"Coping" is certainly the word to use when talking about colic. Colic is rather like the 2½-year-old's negative phase or adolescent acne; that is, one does not cure it so much as endure it. This view may be a little pessimistic, but reading the literature that has been written about colicky babies is somewhat misleading. One might get the impression that colic can be "solved," but it seems to me that, more often than not, the best we can do is to ease the misery until the infant "grows out of it" at 3 to 4 months of age. The instances in which something like a cure is attained are generally cases of true intolerance to a formula or to traces of cow's milk in the milk of breast-feeding mothers. Babies who are fretful because of allergy to a cow's milk formula may have no other symptom than the colicky discomfort. It is not likely to be helpful, but all of us try a change to soy or casein hydrolysate formula in these infants.

The problem of babies who react to the tiny traces of cow's milk in their mothers' breast milk is fascinating. The Scandinavian investigators who first reported this problem claimed that they cured colic in a large majority of breast-fed infants by interdicting all cow's milk products in the mothers' diets. I remember reading this with chagrin that I had not figured it out myself. When I tried the stratagem in my practice, it worked about one time out of four. So, it is always worth a try. The diet must be scrupulously free of all milk and milk products, at least for a trial period of a few days. If it works, many mothers find that they can eat a little cheese or yogurt without causing a sleepless night. A few mothers have found that goat's milk and cheese caused no symptoms. Oddly enough, the problem disappears in a few months, and these babies do not seem to have cow's milk intolerance or other food allergies in larger-than-expected numbers in later life. There is something baffling about all this, and I hope some young practitioner takes on a longitudinal study of these kids.

Aside from diet manipulation, one can attempt to change either the parents or the baby. Changing the parents is pretty much limited to teaching them that infant fussiness is self-limited and nonfatal. Careful evaluation of the baby to exclude significant illness is the first step; sympathetic explanation of the phenomenon of colic (insofar as we understand it!) is the second. I never get very far with the second approach, particularly if the parents can't hear me over the screams of the baby. Changing the baby may be assayed by increased cuddling time (usually already tried before you are consulted), long walks outside (helpful in nice weather), and car rides (amazingly effective with some babies; during the gas shortage in the 1970s, I had one mother who spent her time equally divided between waiting in the lines at the gas station and burning up the fuel in circuitous trips to comfort her infant). Pacifiers are a considerable help, swaddling the infant is occasionally successful (it's the favorite method in Russia), and frequent feedings during the fussiest hours are worth trying. Some mechanical devices are reportedly helpful. One of these attaches to the crib and simulates the noise and vibration of an automobile; I have not tried this yet. The noise of a clothes dryer or a vacuum cleaner is sometimes effective. The tape recording of intrauterine sounds is useful on occasion.

Medicines have a limited place. Some infants are excessive swallowers of air; this should be approached by altering feeding style, but it may also be helped by the generous use of simethicone liquid before every feeding. Rarely, an antispasmodic agent will be useful; one can use belladonna or hyoscyamine. My last resort is sedation. I usually choose hydroxyzine, a minor tranquilizer; I think it has saved a fair number of babies from being battered. The dose is 2 to 5 mg, one to three times a day, as needed to preserve sanity. I know the Academy of Pediatrics has declared alcohol to be the work of the devil, but I still remember my old chief Ed Shaw telling us the remedy handed down to him 70 years ago by his mentor: 1 teaspoon of bourbon, 1 teaspoon of sugar, and 1 ounce of water. When there is nothing else in the house at 2:00 A.M. you might want to remember it, too.

The Family

Within the range of physiologic processes, there may be more stressful times in family life than the newborn period; premenstrual tension and death come to mind. However, there is usually tension to spare in the household of the new baby. If you have time during the 1-month visit, ask how everyone is faring; you will probably not be able to help a great deal, unless you volunteer to do the shopping or the cleaning, but your interest will be appreciated and your question will give implicit permission to complain. At best, the new mother is exhausted; she is probably feeling inadequate in nearly all respects, particularly if her mother-in-law has been visiting. She is worried about her milk supply, wondering whether she will ever lose the extra weight she put on during pregnancy, concerned about paying the bills during a time when she is not working, thinking about child care arrangements to be made when she does go back to work, and maybe feeling a bit stir crazy. Will she ever talk to another adult again about anything but diapers? Often she also feels guilty that she is not happier; after all, isn't this supposed to be the most gratifying time in her life? Having a chance to vent some of this will feel awfully good.

The father is also sleep-deprived, worried about finances, and wondering if his wife will ever lose all that weight. He is also beginning to wonder if she will ever again be interested in sex. The combined pressures of responsibility and sexual imbalance make this period a dangerous one for marriages.

The other kids, if there are any, will have problems as varied as possible. For the older child, say 6 years or older, and especially for a girl, the new baby may be a real delight, much wanted and instantly loved. But not always; sometimes the loss of place in the center of the family universe is the central fact of life, and the child reacts with mourning or fury. It may be well-masked; I recall visiting a new baby at home, where the mother told me how delighted the big brother was with the newcomer. He was so helpful and so happy, she reported. As I was leaving, we heard a rhythmic sound outside the front door; it was the big brother, stamping on the doormat, singing to himself, "Baby go home, baby go back to the hospital, baby go home." For younger children, the baby is generally an unmixed disaster at the beginning. They lose attention from parents and everyone else as well. The grandparents visit and admire the new baby, friends come bearing gifts for the little interloper, and even the family dog seems to like it. Giving token gifts to the older kids is probably a good idea (I always have something in my house-call bag to hand out to siblings), but it doesn't go very far. What the 2- or 3-year-old actually wants is for the baby to disappear.

Fortunately for everyone, babies begin to appreciate their older siblings at an early age. By about 3 or 4 months, most infants think big brother or sister is a charming and fascinating person; often, they can amuse and interest the baby better than anyone else in the family. At this point, the older sibling may begin to see that the baby is manifesting amazingly good judgment and perhaps will not turn out to be a total loss after all. If this is a half-sibling in a blended family, the issues are complex. We'll look at them in the chapter on split families.

Finally, to return to the family dog mentioned earlier, some dogs and cats have practically the status of eldest children, and a couple may worry about the pet's adjustment. I know that may sound ridiculous, but that's how it is. They can be reassured that the long relationship between human beings and our pets has led to a very adaptable population of cats and dogs. They understand what side their kibbles are buttered on and adopt new babies with reasonable grace.

✨ 2 TO 4 MONTHS

After the excitement and exhaustion of the newborn period, the next few months are potentially a period of settling in for everyone. The problem most likely to arise is the mother's return to work. This unhappy pattern has become standard in American life during the last few years. Although there are some wonderful exceptions, it usually means that a highly unsatisfactory day-care setting will be found, characterized by too many babies and too few adult caretakers. The child-care workers can be described only as underpaid, undertrained, and overworked in the vast majority of instances. I am stunned by the collective decision to consign the rearing of America's children to a group of transient amateurs instead of loving parents and other relatives.

The effects of early child care began to be apparent some years ago. I recall the description of one troubled day-care child by a wise psychologist who said, "There's not enough ego there." She commented on the impossibility of giving the kind of love and care in an institutional setting that the human infant needs; mothering is not shift work. Day-care workers come and go; for 8 to 10 hours of the child's waking day, the adults are interchangeable parts in an industrial machine, the day care business. The children pay a price for this in the structure of their being. They also pay a price, and a rather high one, in disease. In the pre–day-care era, the babies in our practice had an average of less than one illness visit during the first year; they now average seven visits for illness. This is the melancholy situation that has become standard. The reaction of the mothers who must leave their infants in generally dubious circumstances and return to work is predictable: they are worried and depressed. The human infant and mother are not designed to be separated in such a fashion or at such an early age, and the mothers know it.

Feeding

This should be a time when either breast- or bottle-feeding is well-established and satisfactory. If the nursing mother has returned to work, either she will be expressing milk when away from home or her milk supply will be rapidly diminishing. Some mothers can maintain enough breast milk to allow mixed-formula and breast feedings; others are less successful. For the formula-fed infant, no changes in feeding are likely to be needed. Depending on the class and caste of the family, there may be a considerable pressure to introduce other foods, especially juices. The history of supplemental feeding in American child-rearing practice is fascinating.

Formula-feeding became popular and practical with the introduction of evaporated milk formula in the early decades of the century. The use of this "modern" innovation suited the mood of the times, and by the 1930s, the up-to-date American mother was feeding her baby with the bottle rather than at the breast. A corollary of evaporated milk feeding was the necessity of giving a vitamin C-containing supplement, and orange juice became the hallmark of mid-century, scientific child-rearing. The equation "Orange juice equals health" was rapidly generalized to "Fruit juice equals health," with a little help from the canned-food industry. My own view is that fruit juices are about as useful as Coca-Cola. They are high-acid, high-sugar, and low-fiber drinks that replace more complete foods, and they are marvelously cariogenic. Children raised on fruit-juice bottles sometimes seem not to have learned that one can quench thirst with water. Parents have so completely bought the notion of the healthfulness of fruit juices that they have great difficulty in restricting their use. I've seen children with anemia, constipation, and declining growth curves as a result of diets dominated by apple juice; their parents were amazed to hear that a quart of juice a day could be interfering with a normal appetite.

The other great triumph of food industry technology over good feeding practices was the fad, now dying out, of the early introduction of solids. By the 1950s, it had become common practice to start a variety of baby solids by the age of 1 month; some enthusiasts advocated even earlier use. It is difficult to imagine what reasons could be devised for this practice, other than a particularly warm regard for the profitability of baby-food companies. One argument was that this taught the infant to use the spoon, as if that were such a desirable skill for early mastery. Parents soon learned that very small infants reacted unreliably to the insertion of the spoon into the mouth and found that adding the solids to the formula worked better. With a generous enough hole in the nipple, you could give a baby nearly anything, and people did. The notion that babies would sleep longer with this fortification was soon disproved by both parental observation and clinical studies. The induction of atopic responses when the infant gut was offered highly allergenic foods was predictable; we saw many instances of dramatic wheat-, corn-, or egg-induced eczema in those days. In short, early introduction of solids was a waste of time and energy at best, and medically ill-advised in any case. Perhaps the fad can best be understood as part of the American distaste for the dependent state characteristic of infancy. Maybe it is a carryover from our frontier days, but there is a powerful strain of American folk belief that fears childhood and wants the child to become a small adult as soon as possible. One sees this in the near-disgust with which pacifiers are perceived, and it is beautifully exemplified in the pretend-adult clothing given to babies. The best example of this I ever saw was a diaper cover made from blue jeans material and designed to look like cowboy clothes.

The eagerness to wean babies from the breast or the bottle is another symptom of our unease with the oral dependency of the young child. In the Sioux culture, children nursed until 5 or 6 years of age; we get upset if a 2-year-old is still nursing. Somehow, the word has gotten out to most of our local families that 5 or 6 months is a reasonable time to start supplemental foods. It is interesting that early solids are still the rule in the black community, with a variety of cereals and sweets offered at 1 to 2 months. If grandma says that vanilla pudding is good for the baby, it is likely to be a waste of time to argue otherwise, but I usually try. Of course, by this age the family is being systematically inundated with advice; not only grandma, but every friend, neighbor, and relative knows how the baby should be fed. Add to that the advice in the shiny magazines and popular books and the glitzy and seductive television commercials; it is amazing that American parents are ever able to hear themselves think. It is also amazing that our contrary advice is ever heeded. Generally, I think, it is not.

I suppose it helps to write down one's Solomonic wisdom for parents to ponder, and I do, and I guess it helps somewhat to repeat important ideas from time to time, but I am not so sanguine that I can compete effectively with the cacophony of other voices. When I hear about "anticipatory guidance" (a pompous phrase, isn't it?), I wonder if the anticipatory guides have any better luck than I do in changing behavior.

Siblings

If you think of it, ask how the other kids are doing. It is usually a little easier at home by now, and the older children may be feeling less worried about displacement. In families with three children, the oldest is often pleased with the effect the new baby has had. It will be apparent that the middle child has been displaced from the darling baby position, and the first-born will consider this appropriate although too long delayed. The second-born, newly demoted to middle child, will also have noted the change and may be reacting in a variety of unhelpful ways. The most common is probably simple regression, and the message to the parents is clear: "If you need a baby around here, I am well-qualified for the job, and you can send the new kid back anytime." So, the middle child asks to nurse or to have a bottle or wets his pants, none of which is likely to impress his parents favorably. Alternatively, he may become depressed, angry, or hyperactive. In any case, the most useful parental responses are simple, repeated acknowledgments of how upset people can get when they feel displaced and repeated evidence that there is still a good place for him in the expanded family. A few minutes once or twice a day with mom or dad (and no baby) can be a great reassurance.

❦ 4 TO 6 MONTHS

Behavior and Development

The personality traits that were hinted at during the first months are becoming increasingly clear by the middle of infancy. Babies who are in constant motion, sleeping all over the crib, scooting and rolling all over the room, and moving from toy to toy within seconds, are rather likely, 3 years later, to fidget during circle time in nursery school;

babies who will become focused problem-solvers may already be engaged in endless analysis of every new toy. There are limits to this crystal-ball-gazing approach to the study of temperament, but it can be helpful to families to have their child's behavior seen in a larger and longer perspective. Families also need to learn what behaviors are simply age- and stage-related. The stranger shyness that nearly always develops in the second half of the first year predicts nothing at all; it is simply the usual response of the child to the realization that the human world is divided into "family" and "not-family." Among American children from nuclear families, the absence of stranger anxiety is fairly uncommon. However, during the 1960s when we saw a large number of commune-reared children, we noted that stranger anxiety was sometimes quite absent. The babies seemed to define adults as pretty much interchangeable parts.

Sleep

By the middle of the first year, most American babies are sleeping for long stretches at night; many are asleep for 8 to 10 hours straight. All American parents are ready for their babies to sleep at least this long, and longer would be even better. Thus the stage is set for one of the first examples of discordance between the needs of the generations. I think this is best thought about in terms of the history of the race contrasted with the present-day realities and expectations of adults. It seems clear that infants and mothers have slept side by side throughout the first few million years of human existence. It is also clear that older children slept next to their parents as a matter of course. The invention of separate beds and separate bedrooms is a fairly recent innovation, and the practice of sleeping away from one's children was probably limited to the very rich until the last few hundred years.

In America today, separate sleeping is expected to be mastered within months, and it is treasured thereafter. Not only does it make possible uninterrupted parental sleep and less inhibited and noisier parental sex, but it serves as a paradigm for the desired growth of the child's independence. Everyone involved with the learning experience benefits, although this is less obvious to the child, who cannot be expected to understand the advantage he reaps in solitary strength. In any event, sometime during the middle of the first year you will hear the complaint that "she doesn't sleep through the night." The age at which steps can be taken to alter this state of affairs depends largely on one's views of the propriety of letting small infants cry for hours and one's fantasies about the effect that the experience will have on the baby. Some years ago, a German mother told me that the practice in her country was to let the babies cry it out in the very first weeks of life; she assured me that German infants slept through thereafter, secure in the knowledge that awakening and crying to be fed were a complete waste of time. This seemed then and still seems to be an awful thing to impose on a newborn, both physiologically and emotionally, let alone the problem for the mother who would awaken bursting with milk by midnight.

So, when do you ask a baby to sleep for, say, an 8-hour stretch? No particularly logical guidelines suggest themselves, but a few pragmatic points may be noted. First, at least one half of all American babies sleep this long spontaneously by 4 to 6 months of age, so it must be reasonably physiological. Second, most parents are becoming increasingly sleep-deprived after half a year of night-waking. A sleep-deprived mother is no great joy to anyone, and her baby will be well-advised to sleep through in order to be rewarded with a smiling and rested mother in the morning. Third, it is amazingly easy to train 6-month-olds not to awaken in the night, and they appear not to hold a grudge. If it strikes you that these three arguments are slender reeds to support pediatric advice, you are certainly correct, but that's life: lots of gray space, little black and white.

Grossman's First Sleep Strategem: The time to teach the baby to sleep through is when both parents are in complete agreement about its necessity. It is too easy for one parent to sabotage the whole process, unless both have suffered enough to face a few nights of misery.

Grossman's Second Sleep Stratagem: The key to learning to sleep through is learning that night-waking is utterly unrewarding; nothing good happens. This means that the baby who awakens is not cuddled, fed, or changed.

Grossman's Third Sleep Stratagem: When the baby awakens in the night, let her know that she has not been abandoned to the wolves.

After a few minutes of crying (the baby's and sometimes the mother's as well), one parent should go to the infant and tell her frankly and firmly that she should go back to sleep. This will presumably reassure the baby that her parents may be child abusers, but at least they are still at home. The parents should be warned that the periods of crying, punctuated by very brief parental appearances, may persist for a remarkably long time. About an hour is usual on the first night, but two or three sets of 1 hour each are not unusual. The second night is easier, nearly always under an hour of piteous screams being about par. The third night is likely to be nearly quiet. Exceptionally, the process may take as long as 2 weeks.

Grossman's Fourth Sleep Stratagem: Parents need to be assured that babies subjected to this program awaken quite happy, even after the most horrendous nights of crying. They are clearly as pleased as ever to see mom and dad, and there are no traces of upset behavior either during the entirety of the training procedure or later. I have yet to hear from my psychiatric colleagues that long-term adverse reactions are cropping up.

Feeding

Introducing solid foods earlier than the middle of the first year is ordinarily the result of external pressure on the parents. The exhortations of friends and family ("Haven't you started to feed her yet?") and the blandishments of the advertisements will often be enough to initiate the process. There are also some very large and very hungry infants whose mothers will tell you that "I can't fill him up with milk." The advice that more milk will indeed fill him up may not be convincing. However, by 5 or 6 months, some of the pressure to start solids may begin to come from the baby. The infant who sits on one's lap during the family dinner, salivating and watching each forkful of food travel from plate to mouth, and grabbing every scrap that comes close—this infant is making a pretty clear statement of readiness to be fed something other than breast or bottle. The baby's judgment may be wrong, but he will doubtless get something to eat, and the venture will probably be successful. Most infants of this age learn easily to manage spoon-fed, pureed foods; digestive problems are fairly rare, although an occasional baby gets completely constipated from baby cereal. The major risk is the induction of allergy from wheat, corn, egg white, cow's milk, orange, chocolate, peanut, fish, and shellfish, and the introduction of these foods should begin cautiously and later.

Parents vary marvelously in their approach to solid feedings. Nearly all are initially enthuasistic, especially about their first-born; feeding our babies speaks to something deep and primitive within us parental animals. The thrill does wear off a bit with subsequent children as we become aware that the first solid foods are a messy chore as well as an exciting rite of passage. Nevertheless, the inner voice of the parent remains: "I feed, therefore I am." This is important; it leads us to feed our young, an absolute necessity, but it gets in our way when the child begins to want control of his food, which the parent may find it difficult to let happen.

What do you feed a baby? I recall the rigid lists we were given by our professor of pediatrics; so many teaspoons of this and that vegetable, fruit, cereal, all dependent on some formula of weight, height, and barometric pressure. It is not all that complicated. First, look at the baby's milk feeding; if it is breast milk or iron-fortified formula, the initial solid feeds are really nutritionally unimportant. Other factors can determine the choices. If it is a low-iron formula, the first feeds should be rich in iron, which really means prepared baby rice or barley cereal. The iron that has been added to that uninteresting-looking powder is very well absorbed, and babies usually like it, especially if it is mixed with formula, breast milk, or pureed fruit. Bananas or applesauce is usually chosen because each is well-accepted and practically never allergenic. If the cereal proves to be constipating, use less and mix in more fruit, especially summer fruits like peaches and plums, either raw or cooked. Other iron sources are meats, which most babies don't much care for at first, and egg yolk, which is something of a mess. For the baby who is already getting some iron, it is still usually a good idea to start with cereal and fruit because it works. An occasional infant prefers vegetables, and that's fine. A reasonable rule is to offer a teaspoon of whatever food is chosen, first once, then twice a day. The volume is increased slowly as the baby's interest and gastrointestinal tract allow. Within a few weeks most babies are taking 2 to 3 ounces twice a day. Another reasonable rule is to add new foods one at a time, at least for the first few months. This makes it easier to determine if any given food is being tolerated; if you give strawberry pudding on Thursday, you will have a hard time ascribing Friday's rash to any one of the pudding's four constituents. Another factor in choosing infant foods is availability. In the American diet, wheat is ubiquitous, and in the form of breads, crackers, cereals, and pasta, it is easily eaten by older infants who have started to finger-feed. Because it is also highly allergenic, one might like to delay its use until about the end of the first year, when the infant's maturing gut might do a better job of breaking it down to a sufficiently digested (and therefore hypoallergenic) form. However, it is basically impossible to keep wheat out of the hands and mouths of American babies.

So, an average baby will start cereal and fruit at 5 to 6 months, vegetables (with or without meat) at 7 to 8 months, wheat at 8 or more months, and the other allergenic foods slowly thereafter. If the infant manifests food intolerance, slow down the speed of new food introductions; there is no hurry. If there are no apparent problems, most babies can be on a complete family diet without any exclusions by 12 to 14 months.

The pureed foods that are used at first can be homemade or commercially prepared baby food. The only commercial food that is really better than homemade is baby cereal because of its excellent iron fortification. Any parent who has a food processor, a blender, or a baby food grinder can prepare superior pureed fruits, vegetables, and meats at a fraction of the cost and with much better flavor than commercial sources. Canning foods inevitably degrades flavors, and baby foods have been made even less palatable because the baby food companies no longer flavor foods with appropriate amounts of salt. Can you imagine anyone wanting to eat pureed, salt-free canned green beans? The notion that it is important to give infants salt-free and sugar-free foods for the few months before they are introduced to the sweetened and salted family diet seems hard to justify. The alternative is simple pureeing of food already prepared for the family—salt, seasonings, and all. Time can be saved by pouring the pureed fruit or vegetables or vegetable-meat mixture into an ice-cube tray and freezing it; this provides a number of rapidly prepared servings.

As the baby develops her ability to reach and grasp, she will usually become interested in starting to feed herself. The variations on this theme are considerable. Some infants not only are excited by finger-feeding, but they want to take over the entire process of obtaining food. They grab utensils from the ministering adult and may refuse any proffered food under adult control. At the other extreme are the babies who enjoy being fed and have no interest whatsoever in taking charge. First finger foods are those that can be managed with the infant's whole hand grasp; puffy rice crackers, graham crackers, toast, celery, meat bones (like chicken drumsticks), and large pieces of soft fruit all are good examples. The parents should be told that they will occasionally have to retrieve a chunk of food from the baby's mouth; it is not a bad idea to teach the Heimlich maneuver, although the risk of aspiration is actually minimal with these foods. **The dangerous foods that are best avoided for the first 2 years are raw carrots, nuts, popcorn, large chunks of wieners and other meats, and whole grapes.** As the thumb-finger pincer grip is mastered at about age 7 to 10 months, smaller pieces of food can be offered. These include dry cereals, pasta, cooked vegetables, cooked and raw fruits, soft meats (such as poultry), and lumpy scrambled eggs. The general theory of solid foods that the parents need to understand is that milk is still the mainstay of the baby's diet, there is no magic amount of solid food the baby must ingest, and the whole undertaking is designed as a transition to the self-fed, mostly solid-food diet of the toddler. This is not a training ground for a Food Olympics with prizes for the largest intake of the most foods.

Safety

Teaching families about safety should really begin before the baby is born, along with the provision of information about car seats for the newborn. After that, safety becomes an issue when the baby starts to become mobile. Timing is crucial; one would like to warn the parents of a risk *before* the baby rolls over and falls off a changing table or a bed. Start to talk about home safety when the baby is about to start creeping. Too long before that time, the topic will seem theoretical and unimportant to most parents; too long after, and the first preventable injuries will already have occurred. This is one area where printed hand-outs are necessary; there is just too much information to give in any other way. We use some original material of our own, we have photocopied a few pages of articles on home safety from a popular magazine, and we use some material from the National Safety Council and the American Academy of Pediatrics. Several types of hazards need attention.

POISONS

Any household chemicals and cleaning substances should be considered dangerous. Some are too toxic to store at all and should be thrown away; these include disinfectants, which are of no utility anyway, and liquid polishes and waxes. Some very dangerous substances like lye and various solvents must literally be locked up. The best rule is to have a fail-safe system with dangerous chemicals up and out of reach and also behind a latched door. Safety latches are available in hardware stores. Every household must have *syrup of ipecac* available in a place known by all of the adult caretakers. Activated charcoal is not a practical material for home use, in our experience. The family needs to know how to report an ingestion: do you want them to call you or the local poison control center? My partners and I ask parents to call us, because we find that poison control personnel tend to overtreat minor ingestions.

ELECTRICAL HAZARDS

The risk of an electric burn from wall sockets is quite small. Even baby fingers are too large to push into those tiny slots. The little plastic wall socket covers are largely useless; babies love to remove them. The main electrical problem is the electric cord, which can be picked up and chewed. The resultant mouth and lip destruction is serious. Electric cords within reach of babies and small children should be attached flush to adjacent walls or baseboards; insulated electrician's staples or heavy tape should be used.

BREAKABLE OBJECTS

The safest approach is to have breakable objects out of the child's reach. The inexperienced parent or the parent trying to hold on to a semblance of a pre-child, civilized ambience may believe that careful supervision of the baby will suffice. "Why, I never let her out of my sight!" This approach fails.

STAIRS

Automatic door closers are easily installed. Sturdy gates are life-saving. Make sure that the baby can't fall through the banisters.

WINDOWS AND DOORS

Safety glass should be installed in any window or glass door that could be fallen against or run into. This is a big and expensive order, but it can be life saving. Sometimes furniture can be positioned to minimize the risk of collisions with dangerous glass, but this is a less certain measure. Children can be protected from falling out of windows by simple devices that limit the size of the opening.

HOT WATER

Turn the heater control as low as possible to minimize the danger of scalds. Ideally the temperature would be 130°F maximum, but this sometimes means that the household runs out of hot water.

HEATING SYSTEM

Free-standing stoves and heaters may need a protective fence. Hardware or building supply stores are good sources of fencing material. Floor furnaces are a hazard in the old houses in our area; we provide a plan for a simple wooden cage to keep the baby from stepping or falling on the hot metal grid (see Appendix C).

OUTSIDE

Gardens need to be free of attractive pelleted snail poison; all garden poisons should be stored in a safe place. The presence of poisonous plants varies depending on your location. Your local county agricultural agent is likely to be a good source of information for you and your families. We frequently look up poisonous plants in one of several textbooks in our office library; the local plant nurseries are useful when you need to identify a leaf in a hurry. A secure fence and gate make outside play possible with less adult supervision.

Making the household environment safe is obviously a major undertaking; recognizing this, I tend to nag. Ideally, I give hand-outs at one visit, discuss the issues and details at the next visit, and follow up some months later. I also use the newborn home call as an opportunity to assess the risks and problems likely to be encountered in a household. With every subsequent child in a family, home safety will need to be reviewed; even in very cautious families, hazards will return as the first child becomes older.

The Parents

In case you have leftover time during a middle-of-the-first-year visit, you might consider asking how the parents are faring. You are likely to hear about a number of problems—financial ones, sexual ones, changes of role, and simple exhaustion. Airing the issue may in itself be a relief for the parent, or it may lead to an appropriate referral for counseling or couples therapy or a parents group. None of these is a panacea, but for an isolated and struggling couple, it is sometimes a marriage-saver.

❦ 6 TO 10 MONTHS

Behavior and Development

As the baby enters the second half of his first year, rapid changes are evident in every developmental area. Most of these changes will be welcomed by the parents; a few will not, including stranger anxiety, increased clinginess alternating with increased independence, and sleep fighting.

Stranger anxiety varies in time of appearance from a few months of age at the earliest to age 1½ years at the latest. Most babies show some caution or fear of adult strangers after the middle of the first year. It is remarkable that this is nearly always limited to adults; the delight and fascination with which infants view children and adolescents hardly waver during the period when most babies are quite shy with grownups. Some infants are selective about the objects of their shyness. They may decide to be shy only with men or people with dark skins or deep voices. There are a few babies who reject all human contact except mother during the height of this phase. This can lead to considerable hurt feelings on the part of fathers and grandparents for a few weeks or months. At about the same time one sees the ambivalence with which the newly mobile infant explores her world. She crawls daringly away, discovers that the adults are no longer in sight, and retreats or wails. She may be brave enough to move out of the room, away from her adult caretaker, but she will object if the adult leaves her for an instant. Some infants become extraordinarily clingy for a while. This passes, just as the shyness with strangers will pass, but it can get pretty wearing on everyone until the baby grows into the next, braver phase.

Sleep fighting is a different matter. Certain babies seem to decide that if they go down for a nap or go to sleep at night they will miss something interesting. They yawn and rub their eyes and appear to try to stay awake by main force. When they are put down, they scream in what sounds like rage, rather than fear or loneliness. If parents can recognize this as an example of infant bad judgment, and enforce the naps and the usual evening bedtime, the babies rapidly agree to abide by the house rules. Unfortunately, in many families the baby stays up as late as the adults; everyone has an infant-centered evening, and the mother and father never have a peaceful, adult minute together. A few years like this can be difficult for a marriage.

Feeding

During these months the infant's diet is gradually expanding to include most if not all the adult family diet. Most babies accept a broad diet with interest and enthusiasm; this helps set the stage for parental concern in the second year, when food preferences tend to narrow. A major change is the increasing proportion of finger-fed food as the baby masters the thumb-fingers pincer grasp. At this point a fascinating process begins which is important as a paradigm for much larger issues. Until this stage the feeding relationship between infant and adult has been characterized by the baby providing cues about his needs and the adult attempting to identify and satisfy these needs. As he begins to graduate to self-feeding, the baby begins to make a different set of choices and gives a new and variable set of cues. It is no longer a matter of "I'm hungry, please feed me." Now it is sometimes "I'm hungry, but I prefer to feed myself." He may show this by turning his head away from the spoonful of food, or by grabbing it in mid-air, or by burying both hands in the plate of cereal. Of course, the simple and appropriate adult response is to increase the availability of finger foods and gradually phase out adult-controlled spoon feeding. For a few months until he can use a spoon himself, the infant can do very nicely with finger foods as the sole solids. But what happens is that most parents react with a combination of resentment and discomfort. Their role is being transformed; they are no longer wholly in charge. Not only is it hard to give up control to the baby, but they are concerned that finger feeding will be inadequate to the child's nutritional needs. "If he feeds himself, it all goes on the floor," the mother tells you, and there is a certain amount of truth to what she says. I like to use this process of uncomfortable transition to alert the parents to the larger question of transfer of power. Here, for the first time, they can see the process of their child's inevitable growth toward independence, and they can experience the concern it evokes in them. We parents have only 18 or so years to turn over full responsibility to a child. The transition to self-feeding is an excellent place to start weaning ourselves from full control of the child's life.

This is also the age when babies are introduced to the cup; a variety of lipped, beaked and covered cups have been devised to make the learning process less messy. Years ago, a wise mother taught me an alternative strategy that bypasses these transitional devices: give the baby a small, unbreakable cup to use at the beginning of his bath. He can practice drinking clean bath water to his heart's content without anyone being concerned about spills.

Safety

I'm sorry to have to mention this again, but it's time. Once again, ask about the safety measures you had suggested at the last visit. What, they haven't been completed? You haven't bought the syrup of ipecac yet? Nag. If you find a more successful approach, let me know.

🎋 10 TO 12 MONTHS

Behavior and Development

Somewhere around the end of the first year, a qualitative leap occurs and one is dealing with a toddler instead of a baby. Actually, a similar change might have been noted a few months before, at the time when the increased social responsiveness and physical skills of the infant transformed him into an older baby. This may sound a little nonsensical, but it is significant. These seemingly abrupt developmental changes continue to occur all through childhood, and through adult life as well, for that matter. We codify them as "stages" and they help us to understand and predict a variety of behavioral changes. The risk of thinking in these terms is that we will be so pleased with the concept that we will try to fit each child and her behaviors into the age-appropriate stage, instead of observing with care the ways in which she may not fit the stage at all. General descriptive statements will not do justice to the variability of human beings.

Having sounded this warning against an incautious use of the idea of stages, I must say that I find them useful. They remind me that development is to some extent predictable, that certain patterns of family struggle can be expected to arise and to subside, and that changes from one stage to the next seem to occur as discrete events. One sees this in learned skills; in one day the child goes from the status of nonswimmer to that of swimmer; the nonreader abruptly gets the idea and becomes a reader. To the observer it seems that a reorganization has happened, rather than an incremental process. Similarly with stages, the baby is all of a sudden a child; the child is all of a sudden a "terrible two." When the family becomes aware that baby has disappeared, having been replaced by a small child, they will be ready to reformulate their expectations and start to respond to the new set of challenges provided by the new person.

Limits

At this point, a major change will be the necessity of setting limits to the activities of their newly mobile and infinitely curious child. The task of teaching children the rules for survival in the home and in society must be met in every culture. For the parents of an intrusive 10-month-old, this generally translates into saying "No!" about 90 times a day. It also means providing a safe environment, which will somewhat decrease the number of "noes." But there will be some situations in which enforcing a limit is a simple necessity. With each child, parents decide what limits they will set. Typically, the rules are most stringent with the first-born. This is largely because inexperienced parents suffer from unrealistic goals and because they have no idea how hard it is to keep kids in line. The accurate complaint of every first-born is, "You never let me get away with that!" as she watches her little sister's mischief go unchecked.

When the first limits are set, the first temper tantrum is not far behind. Temper tantrums are the least appreciated and, I think, potentially the most valuable learning experience of late childhood. When a child wants something forbidden, a sequence of events can develop with considerable pedagogical impact. I want to play with the nice, shiny knife. My mother removes it from my reach. I get furious and scream. My mother comments that she is sorry that I'm angry, but knives are not for babies to play with. I get even angrier, throw myself to the floor and scream louder. Nothing happens! I don't get the knife, no one seems terribly upset that I am so mad, and I get over my anger and find something else to do. If I'm really upset, I may go over to Mom for a hug. I begin to learn that (1) there are limits in my world, some things I cannot do; (2) Mom is still in charge; (3) when I'm frustrated I get very angry, express my anger, and get over it; (4) expressing my feelings is safe, even feelings that are powerful and unpleasant. Well, this ideal scenario is my fantasy of what can be learned through a few years of temper tantrums.

I've gone on about this at length because tantrums are often written about as if they were somehow undesirable for the child to experience. They are certainly experienced by parents as unnerving and often embarrassing. The glares of the lady in the grocery store clearly convey her judgment: "Can't that woman control her spoiled little brat?" There is no protection from the opinions of the grocery store public, I'm afraid. Still, I continue to wonder why writers who want parents to avoid or control temper tantrums fail to appreciate their valuable aspects. I can't imagine a better place to start addressing the subject of frustration and anger than in the family, as a small child. If not then, when?

Setting limits for children at this age involves teaching the child that certain actions are forbidden on pain of parental disapproval. Some babies are wonderfully responsive to these lessons; a mild sharpness of tone or a small scowl will convince an occasional girl (much more rarely, a boy) that a limit must be recognized and obeyed. At the other end of the spectrum are the fairly numerous children who never really seem to internalize rules; I presume that they end up mugging pedestrians or selling junk bonds to widows and orphans. For most kids, it takes 3 or 4 years to build a moderately reliable inner voice that says, "I can't do that."

The parents' best tools in this undertaking are verbal (a good, sharp "No!") and physical removal (to separate child and forbidden object or person). The next step is isolation; children truly hate this, so it works. Fritz Redl, the Viennese psychologist who pioneered psychotherapy with delinquent youth, put it succinctly: To set a limit or punish a child you must get his attention. If he is not somewhat shaken up, he will not notice. Does this sound unduly harsh? After all, we are talking about charming little toddlers. I think that the underlying theory is the same at any age. Get the kid's attention, and make it clear that the behavior is unacceptable and the consequences unpleasant. There are remarkably few alternatives to this method.

The ever-popular American practice of hitting children is often tempting for the parent, especially during the witching hours of late afternoon when everyone is likely to be tired, overwrought, and hungry. In the very short run, hitting works; it does get the child's attention. In the longer run, the disadvantages of corporal punishment outweigh its attractions. Unhappily, it teaches the lesson that big people hit little people and get away with it, not a lesson that one really wants to inculcate in one's children. Furthermore, repeated physical punishment, short of real child abuse, loses its importance; the usual swat on the bottom comes to be discounted by the recipient. Professor Edwards Park is said to have remarked that in order to be effective, a spanking had to be in the nature of a treat; that is to say, something unexpected and rare.

The only other alternative is reasoned discourse, but one discovers that very small children can't be convinced by logical arguments alone. Sometime after age 3, explanations may help a parent to enforce the family rules. If the words are kept simple and reinforced with the old methods of removal and isolation, talking is worth a try. Until then, such attempts are generally useless.

Learning and Play

Toward the end of the first year, the hints of personality pattern that were noted in early infancy are becoming powerfully evident. This is nowhere more visible than in the baby's play. By this age each child has his own personal approach to the world. Clear preferences are becoming evident in choices of toys, style of approach to the household environment, attention span for an activity, response to frustration when an object fails to do whatever the infant had in mind for it, and need for adult attention. The best reason to categorize children along these or other dimensions is to help parents perceive and appreciate the wonderful differences their children express. Many of us begin the process of parenthood with strongly held notions of how we want our children to develop. The feedback provided by the baby can make clear that there are limits, which are set by innate disposition, to the achievement of the parental fantasy. I began to understand this when I gave toy cars and trucks to my first-born daughter; she was perfectly pleasant about rejecting them, but reject them she did. When boy babies of the same age were introduced to her toys, they not only played with the vehicles, but they accompanied their play with motoric sound effects. After seeing this in a few dozen babies, one becomes open to the possibility of sexually determined differences in infant behavior. This was a hard lesson for me to learn as a parent, because it failed to confirm my former prejudice that most differences between boys and girls were culturally imposed. Other parents will have other prejudices and may find it difficult to accept the disparity between expectation and reality.

Feeding

At the end of the first year, most infants are increasingly self-fed; their fine-motor coordination allows enough thumb and finger use for them to eat small pieces of soft table foods. A very few girls will already be using spoons. (Most girls are reasonably adept with utensils by 1½ years, boys by a bit later.) This is an age of slowing growth velocity, and caloric requirements per unit of body weight are dropping. The parent who has been watching the baby eat more and more may abruptly notice him eating less and less. Furthermore, the baby now has quite pronounced food preferences and may vigorously reject what he had previously accepted. He also increasingly demands total physical control of the meal, which automatically excludes all the pureed foods his parents were accustomed to feeding him, and large amounts of his finger food end up in his bib and on the floor. The net effect of these trends is a quantum jump in parental anxiety about food. It is clear to the parent that left to his own devices, the baby will never get enough to eat. This is the time when pediatric intervention is most helpful.

Grossman's First Law of Infant Feeding: Acknowledge parental anxiety, but try to correct it. Parents need to understand that babies know how much food they need; they will not starve themselves to death. **Grossman's Second Law of Infant Feeding: The acquisition of self-feeding skills is a paradigm for the gradual shift of power from parents to child.** It is a safe place for the parent to practice giving some responsibility to the baby, and it is good for everyone. **Grossman's Third Law of Infant Feeding: Help the parents by providing precise information about transitional foods.** The mother who cannot figure out what her baby can feed to herself will have to fall back on what she used to feed to the baby, and a struggle will ensue. Foods that require a spoon must temporarily be abandoned. Finger-feeding babies do best with raw fruits; soft cooked vegetables; small pieces of soft meats such as chicken, hamburger, ham, sausage, and fish; all kinds of pasta; cooked dry legumes; soy bean curd; dry cereals like Cheerios or Chex; and all kinds of breads and crackers. Small sandwiches made with avocado, nut butters, liverwurst, or anything else that will stick to the bread are usually happily consumed. Reheating leftover meat and vegetables from last night's adult dinner is a good idea, since most infants will have their last meal before the grownups are ready to eat theirs. From this generous list, the baby will develop a modest size group of favorite foods; it may appear unduly restricted in terms of adult preferences, but it works fine for the baby. In the diet of the American toddler, the only nutrients likely to be deficient are vitamin C and iron, both of which are added to infant formulas but are absent from the fresh milk that will replace formula in the second year. These are easily supplied: vitamin C from oranges, tomatoes, potatoes, melons, berries, leafy greens, and other green vegetables; iron from meats, eggs, cereals and cereal-based foods, legumes, and nuts and nut butters as well as a little from leafy greens. It is exceptional to need a supplemental chemical source, unless the diet is restricted for medical or other reasons.

❦ THE SECOND YEAR

Behavior and Development

By the beginning of the second year the rate of development of each child's physical skills has become apparent. The range of variation is striking. Some is racial: white children develop more slowly than black children. Some is familial: certain families seem to have powerful patterns of slow or fast acquisition of skills. Some is pathological: slow development can point to disease or underlying disorder. Mostly the variation is simply random and without real significance, except as a source of parental pride or concern.

As we watch growth, we need to keep in mind the limits of this variability. Each skill has its own range of normal. Most babies turn over (at least from belly to back) by about age 6 months, but some soft, fat infants don't manage this until 8 or 9 months of age. Sitting alone can vary from less than 5 months to 10 months. Crawling on hands and knees (or hands and feet) can start by 5 months but 6 to 9 months is usual; some nice, normal kids never do crawl in the usual way. My eldest learned to scoot on her behind while propelling herself with one foot; it worked very well on the linoleum floor of our apartment. (Variation in crawling styles became an issue a few years ago when the peculiar notion was proposed that learning "proper" crawling was a prerequisite to the eventual acquisition of reading skills. One still meets parents who have heard this and need to be disabused.) Pulling to standing is another skill that may be mastered as early as 6 months but may not appear until the second year. The skill to which parents pay the most attention is walking; it can be seen at 6 months and usually is present somewhere around 12 to 14 months, but it can be delayed in normal children to 18 months or more. With all these skills one watches not only the time of acquisition but also the whole pattern of development: physical, social, and intellectual. The baby who is globally slow in all areas becomes a cause for medical concern, whereas the baby who is slow only in physical skills is likely to be a normal variant.

Language appears in an equally variable fashion, and it is sometimes surprisingly difficult to judge. Parents' perceptions of their children's verbal skills may be unreliable; the parents of deaf children can attribute their children's responses to normal hearing, when in fact the child is picking up nonverbal cues. A memorable instance of this in my practice was a family in which the deaf parents, themselves both teachers at the state school for the deaf, were convinced that their deaf younger daughter had hearing. In another family a child was thought to be autistic, when in fact he had severe hearing impairment as a consequence of meningitis. Most infants have some passive language late in the first year; they are likely to understand the names of important people, pets, and objects. Infants begin to use speech actively a bit later; first words may appear as early as 6 to 8 months but more commonly appear just before 1 year. During the second year most speech is in the form of single words; phrases and sentences appear later that year or not until age 2. During this time the child's passive vocabulary is expanding rapidly; even without the help of nonverbal information, the child understands much of what is heard. As part of our observation of the young child, we need to have a general idea of how language skills are developing, but it is necessary to watch both active and receptive speech. I've been thoroughly fooled and unduly worried by very quiet children who hardly spoke for the first 2 or 3 years but clearly understood absolutely every word and sound in their environments. An interesting corollary of this is seen in the bilingual or trilingual family. Kids initially manage two languages quite well; they often ignore a third language. Eventually one usually sees the child preferring the language of peers, and many children in foreign families refuse to speak the mother tongue after a few years, although they continue to hear and understand it.

The child's sense of separateness has begun to appear in the latter months of the first year. Deliberate limit-testing is typical. The baby crawls over to the television, puts a hand on the controls, and smiles wickedly back at the watching parent as if to say, "Are you really going to keep me from playing with this?" In the second year, many toddlers have come to terms, at least temporarily, with the idea of limits, and some of them appear to be having second thoughts about the wisdom of separateness in general. You will see this in 18-month clinginess, a common although not universal phenomenon. The parents may appreciate hearing that this is a passing phase about which they need do nothing at all; just live through it.

Toilet Training

Every little era has its favorite child-rearing problems; in the 1930s and 1940s the central issues were infant feeding and toilet training; now it seems that sleeping through the night has center stage. Why are American families now more relaxed about toilet behavior? I think that mastery of the toilet became less important when automatic washers and dryers became part of most American homes. As long as she had to rinse, wash, rinse again, wring out, hang up, and dry every diaper, the mother had plenty of motivation to teach the baby to use the toilet. Now, the pressure is off both baby and parent. With the availability of disposable diapers, diaper services, and home laundries, one can afford to let the child develop the physical control and psychological readiness needed for toileting.

This new pattern of patience is by no means uniform. The Chinese grandmothers in my practice still start toilet training their grandchildren by the middle of the first year and usually have produced perfect stool control by about age 1—very impressive. I see similar efforts on the part of black grandmothers from the deep South; their methods are different, but they also aim for very early control and often attain it. Early training demands intense vigilance; the baby is scooped up and rushed to the toilet at the first hint of an imminent stool. If the infant is resistant, a titanic battle of wills develops with unpredictable results. I think a substantial number of chronically constipated adults are still fighting grandma when they feel the urge to stool.

At the other end of the stool spectrum are families whose message to the child is that the adults don't care at all when mature toilet patterns are mastered. This does not seem wise; children need clarity about family expectations in an area where baby behavior is different from adult behavior. Otherwise the implicit message may be, "We think that you are still a baby."

It is noteworthy that girls are often more interested in toilet training than are boys. If one provides her with a floor-based potty chair, the 18-month-old may train herself promptly and easily. Then again, she may not, in which case renewed interest may reappear by 2 or 2½ years. Boys are sometimes quite interested in peeing like daddy, standing up next to the toilet; they often enjoy experimenting with urination outside on a lawn or in the dirt. However, their enthusiasm for stooling in the potty chair may be quite limited. Some boys clearly seem to be afraid of the act. One psychoanalytic theory is that they confuse their penises with their stools and fear losing both. I have sometimes suggested that a resistant 2- or 3-year-old boy be given the opportunity to play with a doll, some brown soft clay, and a potty chair to express and work through his fears; the method is infrequently successful but great when it works. However, it would be a waste of time for a boy under the age of 2 years.

Food

Glance at a growth chart and you will see the genesis of most feeding problems of early childhood. After the explosive increase in length and weight of the first half year, the second half year shows a decided deceleration, and the curves really flatten out by age 1. From then until adolescence, growth is slow and more or less steady; it seems to me that parental observations of "growth spurts" represent irregularities of perception rather than changes of size. By the start of the second year, appetite is often diminished; the toddler needs fewer calories per unit of body weight than the mid–first-year infant, so total food intake flags a bit. Coincidentally, the commonly omnivorous food pattern of the baby ("If it doesn't crawl too fast for me, I'll eat it") is replaced by a fastidious concern for just the right food. First to disappear is the vegetable. The sole effect of nutritional education in American schools appears to be that every parent believes life is dependent largely on three servings daily of leafy greens. It is therefore unfortunate that normal, healthy, and thriving toddlers tend increasingly to exclude vegetables from their diets. They usually continue to consume large volumes of milk and juices, and they develop an impressive fondness for cereal-based foods of all kinds. They usually eat eggs and soft meats, and most of them continue to enjoy fruits, but fewer and fewer vegetables pass their lips.

The applicable teaching is **Grossman's First Law of Vegetables: Vegetables are not magic wands for growth.** For practical purposes, the combination of cereals and fruits contains the same general group of nutrients as do vegetables: carbohydrates, indigestible fiber, a variety of minerals, and vitamins A, most of the B's, and C. **Grossman's Second Law of Vegetables: Limit the volume of milk and juice so that the toddler will have some appetite left for solids.** This advice seems self-evident, but it needs to be stated; parents often consider milk and juices to be "beverages," presumably devoid of caloric content and therefore without effect on the child's eating. **Grossman's Third Law of Vegetables: Children are as smart as puppies.** Just as you can trust a puppy to eat enough, you can trust a child to eat enough. The only caveats are that the child is not allowed to fill up on empty calories like candy, apple juice, and potato chips and that appetite is not reduced by ill health or iron deficiency.

Sometime during the second year, the subject of weaning will arise. I've already talked about this in the chapter on breast-feeding. For bottle-fed children, the issues are a bit less complex, since one is not contending with maternal exhaustion, paternal jealousy, and the like. When should a child be weaned from the bottle? Medically speaking, the only problem with continued bottle-feeding is the possibility that an excess of calories will be taken by this route to the exclusion of a balanced diet. Dentally, the only problem is nursing-bottle caries, which can be avoided by limiting juice bottles and by keeping bottles out of the baby's mouth during the night. Developmentally and socially, every culture has its rules about the timing of weaning; the child who continues on the bottle for much longer than the local norm is likely to hear some caustic comments about prolonged babyhood from peers and random, ambient adults. It is, after all, every American's birthright to correct unacceptable variations in the child-rearing practices of others. If the bottle-holding toddler is tough enough, he may simply ignore the pressure. If he is sensitive to his environment, he may decide that he is still being treated as a baby by his parents and wonder why they don't expect him to grow up like all the other kids.

Day Care

Day care for 1-year-olds? The subject would not have come up 30 years ago, but now the day-care revolution is complete. The majority of American mothers work outside the home, and their children increasingly are in commercial day-care centers for many hours every day. The factors that led to this new situation are worth noting, because they affect the way parents feel about day care. First is the degradation of working-class and middle-class incomes over the last decades; a second income is perceived as a necessity by most families. Second is the feminist revolution, which has encouraged out-of-the-house careers for women who in midcentury America would have devoted themselves to the career of mother. Third is the development of the day-care and early-childhood education industries, with their explicit claims for superiority over ordinary home rearing of very young children. The result is a trap. The family needs the money, the mother wants the interest and adult life of a career, and the parents believe that the baby will benefit from life in a group of peers and adult caretakers. The women who are unconvinced and stay at home with small children often feel the disapproval (or envy) of their employed friends. However, the women who leave their children every morning soon discover the discontents of their choice. How do you find a competent and loving person to raise your children for you from 8:00 A.M. to 5:30 P.M. for 5 days a week? Who takes care of the baby when she gets sick? How do you find the energy to be mother, wife, homemaker, and member of the work force, all at the same time? How do you find time for yourself? Whatever happened to relaxed time and play time? What happens to the marriage?

From the child's point of view, if home is bad enough, there is a lot to be said for day care. We all have seen multiproblem families whose children seem to benefit from a well-run day-care program. However, if home is a pretty good place, day care offers a rather mixed bag to the baby. Most obviously, it offers illness; babies and toddlers in day care get sick a lot more often than home-reared children. It offers interchangeable adults who come and go in the child's life. Asking babies to cope with multiple, transient adults is an entirely new phenomenon in human history. We have engaged in an experiment, testing the ability of the infant to develop into a sturdy, socially trusting adult when the infant's experience of adults is that they appear and disappear at random, without regard to the infant's attachment to them. Maybe it will work, maybe it won't. Day care also offers immersion in the world of children, with all that implies: a noisy, undisciplined, exciting, scary, and wonderful place, sink or swim.

All told, I think early day care is a disaster. Kids need a lot of attention from adults who truly care; the likely candidates for the job are moms and dads. If they are unavailable, the very best day care the society can provide should be devised. The stop-gap, commercial arrangements that are common today are bad policy for everyone.

❦ THE THIRD YEAR

Behavior and Development

After the explosive development of the first 2 years, the rate of change slows down and the toddler period of early childhood unfolds. Most 2-year-olds are verbally adept enough to understand the bulk of simple adult conversation, often more than the parents would like to have them overhear. The 2-year-old's active speech will usually be in phrases and some sentences; a few children of this age will be completely conversational with sentences, paragraphs, and all. Play will be increasingly complex, with fantasy productions involving toys, dolls, and stuffed animals. The boys will be involved in cars and trucks. Picture books are favorites, with or without an adult to interpret them. Outside play will involve dirt, sand, water, and wheel toys.

By this age, clear differences are evident in styles of play and activity in general. Some 2-year-olds are intensely physical—running, climbing, and exploring. Others are much more interested in social interaction; they are most content with an adult to mimic or follow or with another child to involve in play. Still others like quiet and solitary play; they look at books or play with household objects or toys. They watch the other children at the park but rarely approach them; they don't head instantly for the slides and climbing structures. This variability seems clearly to be a built-in characteristic; it is sometimes a source of confusion or concern for a parent whose child fails to fit unspoken and usually unconscious parental expectations or desires.

Power

This is the big issue of the third year. Sometime during this year, usually at about 2½ years, the "Terrible Twos" erupt. Here is a piece of folk wisdom that is absolutely real; the family struggles for authority over the lives of these toddlers are predictable and bloody. This struggle is also completely necessary, at least for the vast majority of American children.

The process that seems to be central is the child's dawning sense of its own strength and separateness. It is as though the child has to fight the parents to define personal boundaries. I have often had the image of an assertive and negative 30-month-old child dissecting himself away from his mother and father, trying to discern who he is, as distinct from his previous sense of immersion in and identity with them. Perhaps that is why the fight is nearly always most intense with the mother; the child has, after all, quite literally been a part of her body and her being. However, the fight with father can be just as fierce, especially when the father has taken a large part in the child's care.

The child involved in this struggle is endlessly and inventively assertive, pushing constantly to discover how far her power can be made to reach. The child is annoyingly negative, seeking to prove what she can do by telling the parent what she will not do. This behavior is nearly always limited to the immediate family setting. At day care or nursery school, or at play in the home of a friend, the Terrible Two isn't terrible at all. It is as if the child says, "Why should I bother to fight my friend's mother or my nursery school teacher?

I know that I am separate from them, and I don't have to prove anything."

The response of the parents to this onslaught of aggression largely determines the flavor of the ensuing months. A common pattern for the loving and inexperienced parents of a first child is to retreat, giving in to demands, no matter how bizarre, and placating every whim. The predictable effect is an exponential increase in trouble; having pushed his parents to discover the limits of his power, and finding no clear boundary, the child pushes farther. The analogy of an invading army sending out scouting parties to reconnoiter the enemy's defenses comes to mind.

There can be a number of reasons for parental placating as a way of life. The parents may not realize that the child can understand and accept rules. They may fear the loss of the child's love: "If I don't let him come to bed with us in the night, he'll hate me." Some parents lack a model from their own childhood of loving and firm limit-setting: "When I was a child, the only way they set limits was to hit me." With particularly vigorous limit-pushers, the problem becomes parental exhaustion: "It is just easier to say yes." In any case, the 2-year-old for whom limits are not set becomes more and more demanding and difficult; there is sometimes a frantic quality to the ensuing behavior. It is as if the child says to herself, "My God, who is in charge around here? I'm only 2 years old, and I don't know how to run this family!"

At the other extreme are the parents who respond with anger and rigidity to the child, without considering that perhaps it is time to build a little more power into her family role. A quite punitive and unyielding parental position sets the stage for a long and nasty struggle. I sometimes comment to a parent that we have only about 18 years to turn over complete authority to a child, 18 years to let out rope. The struggles at age 2 are only the first major engagement in a long series of battles for personal autonomy. There will be another predictable phase at around age 4, usually a little less intense than age 2, but tough enough. Again in late childhood, there are the fights about reporting in to mom, about where bike-riding is allowed, when and how to do the chores, who is in charge of television, and so on. The process only escalates in adolescence; the family that fears and attempts to hobble the teenager's thrust for power will have a tough 5 or 6 years.

So, what is the best way for the parents to cope with the 2-year-old on the march? There isn't a "best way," and that is the crux of it. If the process is understood as one of necessary and healthy individuation, most parents can look at the negativism and limit-pushing with at least a modicum of sympathy. If they can then allow an increase in the child's control of her life in some areas, they may be able to maintain firm limits and rules elsewhere. Where those lines are drawn and how they are enforced must be a matter for every family to discover for itself; one family's reasonable rules may be another family's chaos. The tactics also vary depending on the particular child. Some kids make it easy; a clear statement, or even a raised eyebrow, will be enough to tell a timid child that he has reached the edge of his authority. But another child will just about spit in mom's eye rather than submit. With the tough ones, it is usually necessary to choose one's battlegrounds with care. They are so willing to fight about everything that life can become an endless series of time-outs and isolations. Very few parents can tolerate such campaigns of attrition. With these kids, most parents decide to cede power in a number of nonlethal areas. O.K., you can wear your party dress to nursery school, nap on the floor instead of your bed, and bathe only once a fortnight. However, the crucial areas of control had better be kept, and effective methods discovered for convincing junior that he has to live by mom and dad's dicta.

Toilet Training

It is a shame that physiologic readiness to use a toilet develops during the third year. It coincides uncomfortably with psychological readiness to fight mom and dad about everything. The feisty 2-year-old soon understands that his parents really want him to give up diapers in favor of the toilet, and all too often he says to himself, "The hell with it; there's nothing in it for me!" If use of the toilet can be taught by other children, which happens in some societies, or if it is learned in the relatively neutral setting of a child-care center, the child may be able to perceive the act as an interesting opportunity to develop mastery. At home, however, he often sees it as the parents' game, pure and simple.

One way out of this is behavior modification, which some mothers have told me is a fancy name for threats and bribery. I prefer to think simple-mindedly that one can make the use of the toilet worthwhile by linking it with a reward: one M&M if you try to use the potty, dear; two if you pee, and three if you poop. Older children can work toward a goal with more abstract markers: star charts, points that add up to a prize, that sort of thing. Two-year-olds, however, need instant gratification. For some kids, the parents' noisy and heartfelt approval is all they need. That is fine when it works, but don't be surprised by failure. An interesting aspect of the use of behavior-modifying rewards is that the need for the reward rapidly disappears as soon as the task is mastered or the new behavior is established. Somehow the act becomes satisfying in itself.

There are, of course, children who quickly decide that the use of a potty chair or a toilet is wholly incompatible with their chosen lifestyle. They may hide from the adults as soon as they sense an oncoming stool, or they may remain brazenly in view, squirming and straining as they pit their anal sphincters against the smooth muscle of their colons. The child who presses his butt to the floor, or crosses his legs, turning a nice shade of blue in the process, is giving dramatic evidence that he does not want to graduate to the toilet. Generally, the best tack for the parents is to tell the child that he appears to be too young for the toilet, give up the struggle, and return to toilet training at a later date. Perseverance in the face of this intense resistance has a nasty tendency to end up with self-induced, painful constipation; it's a very good problem to avoid.

Daytime control of urine and stool seems to be nearly independent of control during sleep. Only a small minority of newly trained toddlers will be dry at night. Most girls attain night-time control by age 3 or 4 years; boys tend to do so a bit later. If the parents push for a dry bed too early, you can confidently tell them that they are inventing a problem that they do not need. They should be patient; diapers are cheap.

❧ THE FOURTH YEAR

Behavior and Development

By the time the child reaches the third birthday, it is pretty clear who she is and who she will be; this is not to say that personality is set in concrete—but close to it. Of course, the first hints have been evident from a lot sooner than age 3. Once the child is past the newborn period, when the effects of labor and delivery can muddle the picture, temperamental differences begin to become evident. Patterns of persistence with tasks, motor skills and tempo, interest in things or interest in people, general sunniness of disposition or lack of it—all these are well-expressed by the middle of the first year. The developmental processes that result in stranger anxiety late in the first year, clinginess in the second year, and negativity in the third year can hide the underlying personality to a degree. However, by the fourth year all of this is over, and "what you see is what you get."

My sense is that an awful lot of the personality is built-in. I think the observations of the psychoanalysts about infant and child development somewhat misled us into overestimating the influence of the parents. If the kids are psychologically as firmly put together as they appear to be, their ordinary experiences with parents may have less effect in molding personality than the psychoanalysts imagined. The reports of neurotic turn-of-the-century Viennese about their childhoods may not be an accurate basis for understanding everybody else. I'm not saying that parents are unimportant; nor am I saying that a truly batty household is free of adverse consequences for its inmates. I am simply suggesting that the kids come into the world with an impressively well-structured set of personality characteristics already in place. As an amateur gardener I tend to think in horticultural terms, so I tell parents that child-raising is like planting tulips. If you provide a healthy place for the bulb to grow and you feed and water it just right, and you will get a stronger, taller tulip; but no matter what kind of a gardener you are, when you plant a red tulip bulb, what comes up is a red tulip. Parents need to know that their kids are not infinitely malleable, and the parents are not somehow always responsible for the child's problems or, for that matter, his triumphs.

These built-in characteristics become most evident when there are other children in the family for comparison; the differences among kids are far greater than can be accounted for on the basis of differences in parenting. Mothers are often intensely aware of this: "I could tell how different he was from his brother when he was still in my womb." One aspect of these differences is that the fit between a child and her parents can vary from just right, when the parents and the child are rather similar people, to just awful, when the parents and the child are different down to the bone. It can take a long time and some hard lessons before the parents make their peace with the reality of a given child, and decide that she cannot be treated as if she were a carbon copy of mom or dad. I learned a good bit about this from my son Mike. One day, while trying to help him handle a problem, I said, "If I were you, here is how I would handle that." He looked up at me very quietly and seriously and said, "But I'm not you."

Well, anyway, 3-year-olds: they are a nice bunch, by and large. They tend to be reasonable, their verbal skills are good, and disagreements can often be handled with words alone. Generally speaking, they have graduated from the automatic negativism and assertiveness of the preceding year. More often than not, the parents will say, "He's so much fun."

Food

The 3-year-old at the family dinner is the world's best argument for governesses and meals taken in the nursery. There is a powerful, middle-class, American myth that the family dinner is a sacrosanct and peaceful time for the gathering together in amity and good spirits of children and parents. Nothing could be further from the truth. In reality, dinner time is usually the hardest time of day for everyone concerned. The small children are exhausted and usually manic. They were ready for a last meal about 5:00 P.M., long before it was prepared. If they had an adequate snack at that time, they are certainly not hungry when dinner is ready. If they did not have something to eat early, some kids are having a touch of hypoglycemic grumpiness and are too miserable to attend to a meal. No matter how well-timed the meal, few, if any, normal 3-year-olds can sit still long enough to be welcome participants at an adult-type dinner. They want to eat and run.

Furthermore, they generally do not want to eat adult versions of food. The average 3-year-old American child has pretty well abandoned vegetables, he has not yet learned to like salads, he is beginning to distrust sauces, and he sees little excuse for anything much more complicated than bread, cereals, pasta, and apple juice. If he can, he will eat the largest portion of his daily diet at breakfast and spread out the rest over lunch and snacks. Dinner is his smallest meal. Unfortunately, this does not fit well with the adult American pattern of dinner as the largest meal. Dinner is also most likely to be a meat-containing meal, and it is the meal that absorbs the most time and effort in preparation. When a mother says, "She won't eat a thing," she means, "She won't eat dinner." Some feeding problems can be solved on the spot by pointing out that she in fact eats very well, but not in the adult pattern. The remaining difficulties with the myth of the Happy Family Dinner reside in the adult realities of end-of-the-day exhaustion. Parents who have had a hard day on the job are not likely to be the relaxed, interested, wise, and loving people they and their children wish they were. They all could benefit from a revolution of falling expectations.

So, feed the kids early, allow them to leave the dinner table quickly, and grab a little adult time if you can. There will be plenty of time for intense family interaction around the dinner table when they are older.

Nursery Schools

Sometime around age 3, the subject of nursery school arises. Of course many, if not most, American kids have already been in some sort of day care by this age, but more formal preschool is often contemplated as the child toddles into his fourth year. The usual reasons adduced include the availability of more complex and challenging play equipment, formal academic instruction in letters and numbers, perhaps more art and music opportunities, and a bigger social scene. "He'll be bored if he stays at day care another year." There are also the intangibles; I will never forget the mother who smugly informed me that her daughter was attending a nursery school that specialized in ego development. I recall blushing with embarrassment as I realized that my own 4-year-old had stayed at home with her mother and sister and obviously had not been given the priceless opportunity to develop her ego. It took me several seconds to recognize this as utter nonsense.

O.K., what can a nursery school reasonably be expected to do? They are best looked at as transitional places, where the children are introduced to the more structured, school-like settings in which they will be incarcerated until adult life. They will learn to be socialized into component parts of an adult-administered youth culture, interacting with a variety of more or less interchangeable grownups, some of whom may even be well-trained and have the children's best interests in mind. Some of them, however, will be trained very poorly, if at all, and some of the adults, trained or not, will be bored time-servers, long past caring about their charges. In the best and happiest nursery schools the children will learn much about life with peers and grownups; they will stretch their minds, bodies, and voices with new experiences; and they will begin the long road toward independence from their parents. In any nursery school, good or bad, the children also are given innumerable opportunities to cope. Problems arise, toys are fought over, the girl at the next table is a bully, lunches are lost, and teachers have premenstrual tension and low wages. So a nursery school teacher has many chances to help children learn that coping is possible. Improving one's coping skills is probably even more important than learning how to swing from the parallel climbing bars. In nursery school kids can get practice in both areas.

The Three-Year-Old in the Pediatric Office

I've commented that children of this age are generally becoming more reasonable and less resistant to adult direction, and one often sees this in the doctor's office. Seated on a parent's lap, or by himself on the exam table, the 3-year-old may cooperate charmingly with a physical exam. Then again, he may not. In the latter case, it is sometimes possible to use the technique of "paradoxing" perfected by the psychiatrist Milton Erikson. Erikson would help a patient to extinguish an undesirable behavior by demanding that the patient continue and even exaggerate the pattern. When one is faced with a resistant and struggling child, a paradoxical demand can be made that the child scream louder and fight harder. "Oh, come on! You can cry louder than that!" The child will first attempt to redouble his noise, to which one responds by praising the new efforts and urging even higher decibels. Soon he realizes that if he cries and frets, he is obeying your command; he is trapped in a paradox and rather than do your will, he quickly subsides. The odd aspect of this little game is that it is quickly perceived as such, and the most common result is quiet good humor all around. Of course, the trick sometimes fails completely, but it is very satisfying when it works.

❧ THE FIFTH YEAR

Behavior and Development

The best way to think about age 4 is as a rerun of 2½, but with words. More often than not, the 4-year-old will have a period of intensive and annoying limit-testing, most often directed against mother but sometimes generalized against the entire adult world. This usually takes fairly complicated verbal forms; there is lots of name-calling, especially bathroom words. Because the kids have such complete command of language, a common parental error is to suppose that the peace can be recovered and rules kept by verbal appeals to reason. It doesn't work. The issue is not "Does she understand the rules?" but "Who is in charge?" Once again, as at age 2½, parents need to look at the balance of power in the family and decide whether it is time to hand over a bit more authority to the new generation. Maybe it is appropriate to let her choose her clothes for the day or to decide not to share a favorite toy. The formal relinquishment of power in some small areas may be what is needed to satisfy the growing ego. "You're getting to be a big boy now, and you can be in charge of that." These concessions have to be chosen sparingly and well. If the adults retreat too precipitously in the face of the 4-year-old's offensive, the child will continue pushing. He is still looking for clear limits, and he will get frantic if he does not find them.

Oedipus and Electra

Freud was right; kids are really sexual beings. At about this age, even the most obtuse observer will note the unmistakable evidence of children's sexual interest. Four-year-olds are not very subtle about this. The little girl decides to crawl into daddy's side of the bed; the little boy rushes into the bathroom to watch his mother take her shower. Plans are often discussed: "When I grow up, I'll marry you, Mom." Plans are suggested: "I think Daddy should get a little house all his own." Contingencies are thought about: "If Daddy dies, you will still have Adam and Pete and me, but if you die, Daddy is just out of luck." Besides lusting after the parent of the opposite sex, some children of this age are beginning sexual exploration of each other. They may already have learned quite a bit about their own genitals; both girls and boys discover a variety of forms of masturbation. Even the most liberated, modern parents may be taken aback by infant sexuality. "I don't really mind that he plays with himself, but I wish he would keep his hands out of his pants when his grandparents are around." One effective approach to suggest is that genital play is a private matter; it's o.k., but not in public. This is a concept that children of this age seem to understand readily.

Sex play among small and not-so-small children is a great way for them to learn about each other's anatomy, and unlike similar activity at later ages, it is free of the risks of disease and pregnancy. The parent who discovers a giggly game of "Doctor" being played by a happy group of 4-, 5-, and 6-year-olds would be well-advised to back quietly away and let the game and the attendant learning proceed. This may not always be possible; other parents might well object, or a particular child might be thought to be too easily upset. If the children are aware that their game has been witnessed, there is the dilemma of appearing to sanction the children's sex play, something many adults would find quite uncomfortable. Sex play initiated by older children that may frighten a smaller child is another matter, and one good reason why adult supervision of children of diverse ages is a necessity. Parenthetically, this is an important consideration in choosing a baby-sitter. Most, if not all, adolescent boys are too much at the mercy of their sexual impulses to be left as the sole guardians of younger kids.

To return to the subject of the child's sexual interest in the parent, it seems reasonable to help the child give this up. The family that has been happily naked together may need to limit the visual stimulation of shared baths and beds. Doors may need to be closed to decrease the auditory or visual evidence of parental love-making. The child needs to hear that, no, she will not take mom's place when she grows up; she will marry someone else.

School

By now, many if not most Americans kids will have started some kind of school. For the child who has already had a year or two of day care, moving on to nursery school is typically quite easy. It is perceived as simply another familiar group setting. For the child who has been mostly at home, entrance into the world of nursery school can be intimidating: all those noisy kids, all those unknown adults, so much confusion, and no mom or dad. Interestingly, the preponderance of day-care veterans seems to have made it difficult for some nursery school teachers to remember this. The expectations have been changed, and the newcomer is expected to fit right in. This is unfortunate and unrealistic; the process of separation may be prolonged. It can take many weeks until the home-reared 4-year-old can be left without tears and a struggle. He may enjoy the place after his mother has torn herself out of his grasp, but he may cry again when she comes to pick him up at the end of the session.

All this is uncomfortable but normal; most 4-year-olds eventually adapt nicely to the school and its routine. If the adaptation doesn't seem to be developing after the first month or two, it may be best to abandon the attempt. Some children do better with a different transitional place between home and kindergarten; a small play group or a peaceful family day-care setting might do nicely. The entire problem of separation is a nice paradigm for the recurrent questions about child-rearing: How hard should a child be pushed? When should a child's own rhythm of development be allowed to determine the timing of events? Parents may find it worthwhile to have the question of school and separation framed in that fashion. It provides a context for understanding the issues instead of the usual pattern of trying to fix blame for what is perceived as a failure.

The Child in the Doctor's Office

By the fifth year, most kids are fairly happy to visit the doctor. The physical exam can usually be on the exam table; the safety of the parent's lap is not always needed. I try to get a good look at the fundi at this age. Once in a while the necessity to use the minus lenses of the ophthalmoscope tells me that the child is becoming myopic. This is a good age to do screening audiometry with a little transistorized audiometer; our nurses can usually get an accurate test with 4-year-olds. We also do visual screening, either simple distance vision tests with modified Snellen cards or a fairly complete exam with a vision testing machine. The children absolutely love this and often request the "seeing game" at subsequent visits.

Watching the way child and parents interact during the sequence of undressing, examination, dressing again, and leaving for the vision and hearing tests gives some useful information about development and family patterns. Does the parent expect the child to deal with clothes and with the doctor? Does the child play manipulative games with the parent? When I ask the child to leave the room and find the nurse to play the hearing game, what happens? It is a great test of individuation; some kids can't leave, some parents can't let the children leave, some kids race off into the unknown, and some cling and cry. I don't mean to imply that only one way is desirable, although we Americans do tend to greatly value early independence. It is a benign little stress test that teaches me a good deal about the family. If Junior is able to go off on his own, there is a precious opportunity to hear what mom or dad would like to tell you out of his earshot. A nice, open-ended "Well, what else is going on at home?" may elicit interesting answers.

🎋 AGES 5 TO 9 YEARS: MIDDLE-AGED CHILDREN

Behavior and Development

Middle-aged children change so quickly in so many areas and at such differing rates that generalizations regarding development tend to become diffuse or misleading. By and large, this is the age of strenthening ties to peers, increasing importance of the peer cultures (yes, I meant to use the plural), immersion in school, and slowly increasing distance from the family. Boys begin to run in packs at this age. The masculine focus on competitive sports begins to appear. The boys who are not interested in or not adept at sports may begin to be marginalized. On the school playground, boys' games during recess become more and more separate from girls' games. The efforts of teachers to keep a unisex pattern in or out of the classroom become less successful. Girls are beginning to structure complex and often exclusionary friendship groups. The search for a best friend may make for highly charged relationships, and the likelihood that any group of three little girls will remain stable is nil. Someone is always finding herself odd girl out. Next week, it will be someone else.

During this period, some children are beginning to move rapidly into the world away from family. Overnight stays at the houses of friends, the pleasures of team sports, the importance of being with other children as much as possible—all these activities define some very independent kids. Others are tightly bound to the family at home; for them the peer culture has not yet become the center of existence.

The Child in the Doctor's Office

You will see these divergent patterns very clearly when the kids come to see you. The independent extrovert wants to tell you about her illness, about school, or whatever; she races out of the room to find the nurse for her eye test or to go and play on the climbing structure while her parent talks to you. The introvert sits on mom's lap, doesn't want to leave the room at all, and is not so sure the eye test is a good idea. Insofar as the child will let me, I try to increase her role in the medical encounter. Starting with the wholly passive patient role of the infant, the child gradually becomes a cooperative participant in the visit and, eventually, the active source of medical information and seeker of advice. I want to encourage this transition to medical autonomy, so I begin directing conversation and questions to the child as early as I can. Even a 3-year-old can tell me how he likes nursery school, show me where he hurts (more or less), or tell me which ear he wants me to look at first. A few years later, he can give me a pretty good history of an illness, which I will then ask the accompanying adult to expand on. It may be worth noting that some parents find this difficult to accept; the mother who says, "We have a sore throat," has perhaps not yet fully realized that "we" are actually two separate people.

There are some changes in the physical exam for kids at this age. I measure blood pressure at about 5 years, and I get a good look at the flexed spine once a year, at least. Scoliosis screening requires that the children be naked or have nothing on but undershorts. While they stand straight, look at them from the front, the back, and the side, and note the height of the shoulders, the scapulae, and the hips; the size of the space between upper extremities and hips (the "window"); and the curve of the spine erect and flexed. Also note the lower extremity length, carefully estimated with the child lying supine. I find it helpful to shake the child's legs a bit to get them relaxed and centered on the table. Measure the difference in length at the medial malleoli of the tibiae. If the lower extremities appear to differ in length, look for differences in circumference around the thighs and calves as well. Femoral length can be estimated with the child sitting erect, legs over the edge of the table: is one thigh longer than the other? Lower leg length is estimated with the child prone and knees flexed to 90 degrees: is one foot higher?

If there is a hint of scoliosis, measure the maximum height of the rib ridge with a nice little device called a Scoliometer; it is like a small carpenter's level. Also measure back straightness with a plumb line held at the C7 spinous process. You will find dozens of kids, mostly girls, with a little scoliosis that never amounts to anything. They are neurologically normal, have no symptoms, and need nothing but observation. If there is a considerable leg length discrepancy, say over ½ inch, and increasing scoliosis, a firm ½-inch pad glued inside the shoe on the short side is probably a wise idea. When should we get a radiographic evaluation? I don't know any hard and fast rule, but generally I order films when scoliosis is increasing, when the size of the ridge is more than about 8 degrees on the scoliometer, and if there is a family history of scoliosis.

I mentioned that the child must be disrobed at least down to underpants for the back exam. The issue of clothing and modesty is worth exploring a bit further. From the time of the first physical exam of the infant, I think the examiner owes it to the child to be complete and thorough. This truism implies that one will remove the diapers of an infant or a toddler, and that the underpants of the child or adolescent will also be shed during a complete physical exam. This is more easily said than done. For one thing, you will not always really want the infant's diapers removed, because the attendant mess will call for someone's attention, and that someone might just happen to be you. On the other hand, I recall my old chief Ed Shaw saying that it didn't make much sense to ignore the one quarter of the baby under the diaper.

Sometime during childhood the abrupt appearance of sexual modesty may make the child uncomfortable with genital area examination, and a certain amount of resistance can be anticipated. This should not be handled with brute force. Discussion and explanation may be necessary and will nearly always suffice. I think this problem is minimized by making under-the-underpants exams absolutely routine and matter-of-fact throughout childhood. The meta-message to the child is that the genital area is a part of the human body that gets examined like any other part; it doesn't offend or frighten the doctor, and the child need not be frightened of that part of his own body, either. The current hysteria about child abuse has given this subject a difficult twist. Because of what seems to me a completely ill-conceived notion, a substantial number of children are systematically inculcated with the lesson that adults are potentially dangerous. The lesson is doubtless true, but the idea that little children have a significant role in protecting themselves from sexual abuse is fatuous. It is our job as adults to protect kids and their job to grow up with as much trust in their fellow beings as is possible.

School

School is a big enough subject to require its own chapter, which it gets later in the book. A couple of comments seem to fit here. The first has to do with the question of time of school entrance. The standard American pattern of kindergarten at age 5, or thereabout, began when there was no such thing as nursery school; kids stayed at home with family adults and children and the neighborhood kids, if there were any. The kindergarten was designed to be just what the word says—a garden for children, where they could learn to enter gradually and gently into the adult-organized world of schooling. Now, however, the children arrive with wildly divergent group and school experiences, ranging from years of group day care and academically pushy nursery schools to life on ghetto streets, taught by peers and passers-by. In some school districts the preponderance of academically experienced children has led to the introduction of what were once first-grade learning materials into the kindergarten classroom. This has had the unexpected effect of turning a substantial group of 5-year-olds into instant school failures. A lot of kids, especially boys, are not at all ready to read and write at this age. So the savvy parents keep their boys out of kindergarten until age 6, or they let them repeat it after a year of struggle. The older boys are then more likely to settle down to learning, but they are now a year older than their classmates. This is a small but significant difference, and it gives the older boys a permanent advantage in the one area that counts in the little boy culture, namely, sports. Conversely, the boy who was successful as a 5-year-old in kindergarten is presented with a permanent and unearned disability: simply because he is younger, he is highly unlikely to catch up to the older boys' prowess in sports, especially if he happens to be small or slow in physical maturation. Eight or nine years later, he will be prepubertal at a time when his older classmates are sprouting in all directions; this is a social disability of some magnitude. None of this is end-of-the-world in importance, but it needs to be balanced when a parent wants your opinion about early versus late school entrance for junior.

Because girls are much more likely to be able to do academic work at age 5, the issue will come up less often with them. When it does, keep in mind the various disadvantages of being out of step in the girls' peer culture. Sports matter much less for American girls; the sources of status are academic success and popularity (with other girls at this age and with both girls and boys during later childhood and adolescence). If you are older, you may get leader status by virtue of your better-developed social skills; but when adolescence arrives, you leave your sister schoolmates behind as you develop new interests and new body parts. Being the oldest girl in your class can be a lonely business in junior high.

The wide range of school readiness exhibited by 5- and 6-year-olds leads to some interesting problems in the early diagnosis of learning disability. Ideally, one would like to have a precise and sensitive test to point to the kids who are dyslexic or hyperactive, or both. Well, there is no such thing. It takes the combined efforts of teachers, parents, and pediatricians to pick out these problems, and none of these groups is particularly well-trained for the task. For example, teachers may be misled by class and ethnic patterns. By middle-class white standards a lot of ghetto black boys will look hyperactive. The teacher may equally be misled by a quiet, well-behaved, and bright girl who sits without complaint in class, never drawing attention to herself or to the fact that her dyslexia is causing a child with an I.Q. of 150 to do average work. Nearly all teachers are also overworked and overwhelmed by the large class size that typifies American classrooms. Since teachers do not tend to think in terms of diagnosis, their observations serve as a screening, early-warning system at best. Parents often suspect problems in this area. Needless to say, they also lack training, but as is always the case, a parent's questions about a child's school work or behavior patterns bear careful hearing. As is so often true in primary-care practice, the pediatrician's first role is to make some management decisions. Is the child active or hyperactive? Is his letter reversal pattern within the normal range for his age? Is there a ghastly family, neighborhood, or financial problem, of which his school performance is just a symptom? Does he have a tired, time-serving teacher who just cannot bear a noisy little boy? In short, does this situation deserve a careful, potentially upsetting, and certainly expensive workup? In the later chapter on schools, I'll look at what to do next.

The Over-Scheduled Child, Sputnik Syndrome, and Baby Burn-out

When I started practice in a suburban university town in 1959, I was amazed to discover a previously undescribed form of child labor, the over-scheduled child. These were kids and adolescents who left for school early to take the pre–regular hours elective class (music or art or a foreign language, usually), stayed late for another elective, then went to (1) dance class, (2) art class, (3) pottery class, (4) religious school, (5) Chinese language and civilization class, (6) baseball, (7) swimming, and on and on and on. At first I reacted greedily: I wanted all of that richness for my own 4-year-old. Slowly I began to notice that the kids were, by and large, a mess. For years they had worked 8-, 10-, or 12-hour days at becoming skilled and wise, and by the time they hit high school they were ready to light up and drop out. That "Sputnik" generation, raised to catch up with the Russians and to be sophisticated, worldly, and talented was badly served by the anxiety of their parents and teachers.

Today, in our suburban university town, the opportunities for an enriched education outside of school hours remain as seductive as ever. Now, of course, we are supposed to catch up with the Japanese. The main difference I see is that sports are being pushed harder, and the schools no longer have early and late classes. Many of the kids are still scheduled to within an inch of their lives. The eagerness to push the children as soon as possible onto the treadmill of too-busy adult life is fascinating. Parents who complain bitterly that they never have time for themselves or their family carefully arrange their kids' lives so that there is no time for the kids to relax or be with their parents. Do we grownups resent and hate childhood?

❦ PRE-TEENS

Behavior and Development

Medicine and bird-watching have in common the development of skill in pattern recognition. The bird-watcher learns to look for the telltale combination of markings, flight pattern, or song; the physician becomes sensitized to the grouping of signs and symptoms: the same skill. Pre-teen kids will provide you with the opportunity to note some striking patterns in human development. As they grope their way from childhood toward adolescence, some children fall into clearly recognizable types, as easily discernible as wrens are from blue jays.

The Organized Girl is a fine example. Children in this category often begin to show themselves in early childhood by the way they line up their dolls on the shelf. They are generally choosing their own clothes every morning by the time they are about 3 years old. In school they quickly learn the rules and are teachers' helpers instantly. By the time puberty is starting, they have taken on significant household responsibility and can be seen calmly evaluating their mothers' methods of cooking, cleaning, and child-raising, with the implicit judgment that they can and will do it all better. Some of their mothers do not take kindly to this. Among their friends, these girls are the leaders and idea sources. They edit the school newspaper and run the fund-raisers. All this talent may be wrapped up in a charming personality package; then again, it may not.

The Teenie-Bopper is different. These children look at adult patterns of life with an attitude between disinterest and loathing. They are early converts to the styles of the adolescent. They are listening to hip-hop or punk or heavy metal before they are out of grade school; they demand the correct brands of all consumer goods; they know which idols of popular culture are still worth idolizing and which are on the way out. The female Teenie-Bopper is in a hurry for her first training bra and for real boy-and-girl parties. The male of the same age may find himself somewhat out of his depth with this aspect of Teenie-Bopperism, although the rest of the teen scene looks awfully good to him. His parents may wonder why so many little girls keep calling him up; he may wonder about it himself.

The Reluctant Scholar has often surfaced by this age. School may never have been much to his liking from the start; by the end of grammar school, he (usually he rather than she) has begun to dig in his heels. He lies to his parents about homework ("She didn't assign any tonight") and to his teacher as well ("I lost the binder"). These children are not, for the most part, stupid, brain-damaged, or emotionally disturbed. Their interests and academic life are simply immiscible. They need a nonacademic environment as soon as one can be arranged. It is a profound mistake to believe that every child and adolescent is best served by the same curriculum. By the start of junior high school, this becomes painfully obvious.

The Boy Who Does Not Like Sports is a small, sad category. Whether the disability is muscular, hormonal, or temperamental, he has little interest and less skill in the playground activities that enthrall his sweatier peers. This may already have become a sore point at home if his father equates masculinity with Monday-night football. Finding a substitute activity can be a big help. This might be an unusual but socially acceptable sport (e.g., table tennis, swimming, bike racing) or a nonsport area for competition and success (e.g., chess, photography).

In general, the pre-teen group is notable for a quantum jump in independence from the family. An annoying sign of this is the style of speech that parents of an older generation termed "sassy" and modern parents are likely to call "smart-ass." This is in no way a recent phenomenon; the erosion of respect for one's elders has been noted and regretted for several thousand years. However, it does seem to be particularly virulent in an age when most of the rules of verbal interaction between the old and the young have been abandoned. Parents are appropriately taken aback by the snotty know-it-alls who abruptly appear at the dinner table. My own view is that the newly sensed independence that underlies the disrespectful speech can be quietly appreciated, but the adults should take the opportunity to restate family expectations about the proprieties. During the tug-of-war that will be developing during the next few years, the parents need to be as clear as possible about where they remain in charge and where the kids can take over. Guidelines about manners within the household are a good reminder during this transition.

Sex Education

It is often about this time that parents will ask for guidance concerning sex education: what books to provide, who should talk to whom, or whether perhaps the doctor would like to do this during the next checkup visit. Unfortunately, the parents are usually too late. It seems to me that the most important parts of sex education concern the way people relate to one another, the way the human body is viewed, and the power relationships of the sexes. Is human interaction marked by consideration and respect, or do people exploit and dominate each other? Does the family's balance of power teach that both sexes are to be respected as important, or that one sex exists to serve the other? Is the child taught that the genitals are dirty or shameful and that masturbation is evil, or that the body is a wonder and a joy? All of these lessons are the foundation of the adult's sexual functioning. Teaching the 12-year-old about breasts, menstruation, erections, and all the rest is fine but rather after-the-fact.

Still, somebody has to teach the anatomy and physiology of sex, and parents will want some guidance. You will need a little familiarity with the lay literature; invest an hour at your local library or bookstore to find out what is available. The reference librarian at the public library can help. There are the publications of the American Academy of Pediatrics and the American Medical Association in inexpensive booklets. Planned Parenthood is another source. In many school districts, sex education is thoughtfully and fully incorporated into the curriculum of primary and secondary schools. Oddly enough, the kids who need the most home education in this area are likely to be the ones who attend private schools where sex education is frequently ignored. Parochial schools are wonderfully variable; some focus wholly on "thou shalt not," and some really teach.

When the parents embark on this enterprise, it will pay them to have read the material before giving it to the kids; most adults need a quick review of the facts to be able to answer a question with any accuracy. The children often react to the parents' sexual pedagogy with embarrassed avoidance; the parents may have to persevere over a long period of time. They will not enjoy the procedure. Eventually, in a substantial number of families, sex can become a true subject for discussion, instead of the Great Secret, second only to the family finances as something never to be talked about. I will never forget my daughter, age 15, sitting down on the rug between her mother and me one Sunday afternoon and asking whether we thought it appropriate for her to start having sex with her boyfriend. I thought it was wise of her to consider our opinions, and I thought it was wonderful that she trusted us enough to talk about the subject. No, I won't tell what we said.

Pushing Kids: Music Education as a Paradigm

All these issues—sassiness, independence, sex—are linked by the question of how much the parent should stay in charge of the child. In many instances, this devolves into a struggle between the parent, who wants the child to do something, and the child, who doesn't want to do it. Whether it is using the toilet at age 3 or working harder in school at age 13, the parent must often decide whether, when, and how to push. A classic example is teaching music. I had not been long in practice before noting the common and melancholy sequence of failures in extracurricular music education. The mother of the bright little 7-year-old reports happily that he has started to take piano lessons; the teacher is said to be impressed by his enthusiasm and talent. At about age 8 I ask how the music is going and learn that the lessons are proceeding, but under duress; he resists practicing, and the teacher wants the parents to insist on half an hour a day "so that he can make progress." At about age 9 I ask about the piano, and the mother grimaces and says, "We gave it up; I told him we were not going to pay good money for lessons when he refused to practice." In short, if one defines music as a drudgery imposed by the teacher and enforced by the parents, one can pretty well predict that a self-respecting child will decide that there is nothing in it for him.

The problem here lies in the music teacher's assumption that continual practice is the only road to proficiency. It is as if the teacher of pottery insisted that the weekly lessons in the studio were useless unless the child took a bag of wet clay home to work on every day. In fact, if the teacher can relax about practice when the child wants to do other things, a weekly music lesson can work very well indeed. Progress will be slow, no doubt; this is not the way to make Horowitzes. However, music will not be abandoned. If the teacher can accept this without feeling insulted and the parents can understand that the choice is between no musical education and a leisurely one, this laissez-faire approach can keep children learning and loving music. It may also serve as a valuable model when other issues arise between adult goals and a child's sense of what is right for him. Sometimes we have to listen to the child.

🦠 ADOLESCENTS

Who Is My Patient?

We had better ask ourselves this question regarding teenagers because it has to be clear to everyone concerned—the kids, their parents, and us. I guess the best answer continues to be "the whole family." The difference between this and earlier ages is that divergences between the needs of the adolescents and the adults become more frequent and obvious. So we have to set out some new ground rules. Here are mine: (1) Whenever possible, I want to see the adolescent without the parent being present. If the parent is there, I want to deal with the adolescent as much as possible without a parental intermediary. This may sound as if I am treating the parent as some sort of adversary—either of mine or of the teenager—but that is not the case. I try to structure the visit to teach autonomy and self-reliance, but I continue to respect the parent's authority and role. (2) Sometime during a patient's adolescence I tell the kids and parents that I consider whatever I am told to be privileged information; I can be trusted to keep confidences. This rule does not apply if I consider that danger to anyone will result. (3) In order to be useful to the family and also to get a more rounded picture of an adolescent's life, I ask the parents to come in once a year, without their child, for a talk visit. About half the parents do this. When the parents are divorced, arranging separate talk visits for each parent is ideal, but I find this impossible. Having both divorced parents at the same visit is interesting but excruciating for everyone.

I suppose a few years of training as a family therapist would be helpful in this situation.

The Physical Examination

A yearly physical examination of teenagers gives one the opportunity to pick up unexpected problems, like hypertension or scoliosis, and problems known but unacknowledged, like acne. It also lets the examiner do some teaching about sexual and physical development and what can be expected. I like to make informal predictions about eventual height and likely age of menarche, subjects in which adolescents are invariably interested. Late in adolescence, I sometimes tell boys about self-examination for testicular cancer and girls about breast cancer. This information must be timed with some care. If a teenager is already hypochondriacal and anxious, I tend to put off this discussion as long as possible.

I have never managed to solve the various problems of incorporating pelvic examinations into the routine of wellness care. There is really not enough time in my 30-minute well visit for a first pelvic plus the rest of the physical examination and an interval history. I also want to give the young woman some advance notice that her first internal genital exam is going to be done; it does not seem like something to spring on her half-way through the visit. Asking her to make a return appointment for the pelvic is not always successful either. More often than not, a first pelvic will be done when she has a specific symptom requiring it, and quite often a visit to Planned Parenthood or a local gynecologist will be the occasion. In general, however, I think her pediatrician is the best person for a first pelvic. In her regular doctor's office the young woman does not have to cope with new people and new surroundings. The exam is less likely to be threatening and more likely to be perceived as a logical extension of previous medical care. The pelvic can be done using a regular examination table, without stirrups. Lying with her buttocks at the end of the table, the girl flexes her knees, abducts her hips, and keeps her feet together. I don't use a drape because I want her to see and understand the examination, and pretending that a pelvic is some kind of surgical procedure requiring extra linens seems quite bizarre. During the exam,

I explain exactly what I am doing and what I find. We use disposable plastic specula which feel less cold and unpleasant than steel. Most young women find the exam easy, not particularly uncomfortable, and less embarrassing than they had anticipated.

I know my malpractice insurance carrier will not want to read this, but I don't have a nurse chaperone pelvic exams. These are kids I've known forever; they trust me and I trust them. The presence of a third person to protect one of us from the other would strike both of us as peculiar. With a brand new patient a nurse chaperone does make sense, and, obviously, the situation is quite different in other settings, such as hospital emergency rooms and public clinics. If the mother has come along to the visit, the question of her presence during the pelvic should be up to the girl herself. Most often, girls prefer to have mom out of the room.

Personality Development in the Teens

Despite the myths of the media, adolescents cannot be characterized in any simple fashion. This is worth mentioning to the parents of pre-teens, many of whom live in dread of the terrible teens. I recall the comment of a physician friend who had 6 teenage children; he said it was awfully noisy but wonderfully exciting. Within the limits of this generally accurate description, there are a few recognizable patterns.

✳ Girls often signal the approach of puberty by a distinct increase in volatility of mood. Easy tears and easy rages may upset the family and puzzle the girl herself, who may wonder whatever is happening to her. What is happening is hormones, and it will take her a while to learn to live with them. As adolescence progresses, she is likely to be in conflict with her mother more and more. The process of becoming a woman in her mother's house implies a certain amount of rivalry between them as the girl separates herself and defines herself in a new way. This is often an exceedingly painful process for her mother who finds her daughter increasingly distant and hostile. It is a kind of re-run of 2-year-old negativism with strange sexual overtones. The adolescent girl may stay quite close to her father during this early period. But as she begins to have sexual feelings for her peers, starts to date, wants more freedom to come and go as she pleases, and borrows the family car, the relationship between father and daughter can become quite tense. It can be difficult for dad to accept the reality that his little girl is not so little any more, that, in fact, she is a sexual being with her own agenda in the world. By the late teens, a substantial number of girls have made their peace with mom. It turns out that there is room for two women under one roof and both the mother and the daughter can accept that they are different and separate people.

Personality changes in adolescent boys can be summed up in one word: testosterone. This does not always mean trouble, but it does imply a certain amount of brisk rearranging of family processes and power. As he approaches the mid-teens, the adolescent male is often becoming fairly restless. He wants a longer leash or no leash at all. He continues to shift his interests and allegiances away from home. School may appear wildly irrelevant to his world. As he feels his growing strength, his behavior in the family may become decidedly less compliant and more challenging. His parents will have a nice task deciding how fast to loosen controls and how much effort it is worthwhile expending to maintain the old rules. Occasionally none of this happens at all. The growing young man remains contentedly ensconced at home, does not challenge anybody, continues to be involved with school, and is perceived by his parents to be an ideal teenager. I worry about these kids. Why are they not moving toward independence? Is it too frightening? Is the family constellation so fragile that the boy believes that his growth would shatter it? Whatever the reason, failure to assert some independence at this age is a symptom to be studied rather than a situation for the parents to enjoy. The period of male rebellion seems to be quite prolonged for many of our young men. While a substantial number of young women apparently work out their new relationships with their parents by the end of the teens, my impression is that this process is extended into the twenties for many men. Perhaps it is related to the common situation of endless schooling that delays financial and vocational independence. In any event, the young lions challenge the old lions again and again.

The Hypochondria of Change

One way to deal with adolescent change is to worry about it, so some kids fasten all their anxieties on their bodies. They note every borborygmus, are cancer-phobic about every mole, and even consider avoiding no-calorie soft drinks because of the chemicals. This syndrome can be recognized in its pure form when the teenager appears for a brief illness visit and pulls out a little list of complaints. You will have to deal with the whole list, and then, if you have the time and patience, consider talking a bit about how people can get concerned about all sorts of small matters when big changes are taking place.

A common complaint at this age is chronic fatigue. Medically sophisticated families will have kids who are sure they have the recently described chronic fatigue syndrome, and perhaps a few of them do. A tiny proportion will have associated signs or symptoms suggestive of hypothyroidism; I have found one such patient in the last 30 years. But the vast majority will fall into one of three groups: the excessively busy, who need more sleep and fewer activities; the anxious; and the depressed. Neither of these latter two groups can be dealt with rapidly or easily. It may take a fair amount of time to help them learn that their tiredness is a mask for other problems. Sometimes a few talk visits of 20 to 30 minutes is what they need to regain a perspective on their lives; rarely, they will be interested in formal psychotherapy, but this is usually resisted with considerable vigor. Adolescents are often sufficiently self-absorbed to be fascinated with simple techniques of self-study. I sometimes suggest that a diary will be useful to clarify issues and feelings. For those with a literary bent, I may suggest that they write letters to themselves about their problems. Another technique is to have them draw pictures about problems. The concept of sub-personalities, representations of the varying needs and tendencies within one's self, can be used. I will ask the teenager to draw a cartoonlike picture of each of the competing sub-personalities in order to become cognizant of the inner complexity and, eventually, to accept the reality of competing parts of oneself. Teenagers in general are quite resistant to entering into a formal psychotherapeutic relationship, but the trust they already feel toward a familiar pediatrician can make these gentle methods acceptable.

Food

Anorexia and bulimia are now epidemic among adolescent American girls. The pure anorexics will be obvious. The bulimics will be hidden, and you will be surprised and chagrined when one of your apparently healthy patients tells you that she has been making herself vomit for the past three years. More about this painful problem in social and psychological pathology in a later chapter.

The usual problems of normal teenagers' diets are deficiencies of calcium, iron, and vitamin C. A substantial proportion of American kids grow up drinking soda pop and miscellaneous juices instead of milk. Fortunately, some of them quite automatically begin drinking milk when their growth spurts start, a nice example of the wisdom of the body. However, some bodies are pretty dumb, and nutritional counseling is needed. For practical purposes, calcium is available from milk and milk products and not much else. It is possible to devise a diet with enough soybean curd, nuts, oatmeal, and greens to provide a modest amount of calcium, but not nearly enough for optimal bone growth. Calcium supplements are the best answer although they tend to be constipating and the tablets are rather large. Generic calcium carbonate or calcium phosphate (dibasic or tribasic) are inexpensive. Calcium-fortified orange juice is another alternative. The "fresh" soy milks sold in dairy cases are not rich sources of calcium and should be avoided.

Iron is a major problem for the menstruating girl who loses iron with every period. Many of these kids take a minimal caloric intake in order to control their weight. If they also happen to be inactive rather than athletic, their caloric needs are quite modest, and it becomes difficult for them to get enough iron from a typical diet. Iron-deficiency anemia results. During childhood, enriched grain products (breakfast cereals, bread, pasta) are major sources of dietary iron. If the adolescent skips breakfast (most do) and avoids bread, she will have to get by on the iron in meat and eggs (currently out of fashion), nuts, and dark leafy greens (never in fashion).

Vitamin C is certainly not hard to get in the American diet, but a substantial number of teens manage to avoid it. It is worth mentioning to them that the sources are oranges, orange juice, tomatoes, potatoes, dark leafy greens, summer fruits (especially berries and melons), or, failing all of these, vitamin C tablets.

Sex

Am I the only pediatrician who finds it difficult to talk about sex with adolescents? Somehow I doubt it. I know that all the books and articles on the medical care of teenagers tell me to raise questions about sexual activity, preferences, safe sex and contraception, and in the best of all possible pediatric worlds I'm sure I would. But in the real world I don't push this very hard. Not that I consider sex an unimportant subject; in one form or another, it figures in well-child visits from infancy on. The effects of nursing and parenthood on the sex lives of the parents, the Oedipal behavior of 3- and 4-year-olds, the questions of sex education timing and content all through childhood—all these subjects are grist for the mill. But what is the practitioner's role in exploring the sex lives of adolescents? I feel constrained by my sense that this is terribly private behavior from which the adult world is largely excluded. I suppose that, given the proper questions and enough time, one might find that a significant number of kids would like to discuss sexual concerns. What I have done instead is to ask a few questions about menstruation, birth control, and dating. I want the kids to know that these are o.k. areas to talk about, but I also want them to know that I respect their privacy.

Drugs

Another uncomfortable area. Is there any point in asking directly about drug use? My assumption is that teenagers will generally tell me what they think I want to hear, so I don't ask. Instead I ask about drug use at their schools and among their friends, trying to get a general idea about the importance of drugs in the peer environment. This will occasionally lead to significant exchanges of information, and it does help me keep abreast of the changing patterns of drug use in the community.

Graduation from the Pediatrician

Back at the turn of the century, we pediatricians first defined ourselves as baby doctors. Then we expanded our role to include other children and young adolescents, and now we find ourselves taking care of young adults as well. What makes the most sense for us and for the patients? It seems to me that most kids do well to stay with a pediatrician through adolescence. We are focused on the problems of growth and development and the diseases of youth. We understand the issues of education and independence that concern people in their late teens and early twenties. And until the young person is out of the family home and launched into the adult world, he probably does best in a familiar pediatric setting. Of course, some teenagers become uncomfortable in an office full of babies. I know that some of our burly, bearded young men are embarrassed when the nurse mistakes them for fathers rather than patients. But most of them stay with us until independence and employment. I tell them that they are welcome until they get a master's degree or get married, but I've been known to make temporary exceptions to both conditions.

❧ CHAPTER 11

Split Families

One of the least happy aspects of pediatric practice is watching families come apart. Sometimes the disintegration of a marriage is prolonged and public. One has the opportunity to offer advice about family therapy or marriage counseling, and sometimes the advice is taken and is useful. More often, in my experience, the problems have been successfully hidden from me; I learn about the impending or completed separation in a burst of parental tears at a well checkup or an illness visit. Ours is a psychiatrically aware community, and many of these couples have already worked with therapists in a failed attempt to solve problems. Despite that, I urge the parents to consider psychotherapy during the period of separation and divorce. There are a myriad of practical problems to be dealt with when parents separate, and the heavy weight of anger, sadness, and confusion surrounding divorce makes clarity difficult to attain. A skilled therapist can help parents sort out the best solutions, even if the marriage cannot be salvaged. Many of these problems will involve the children, and if they are old enough, a family therapy approach may be ideal. At any age children will be confused, frightened, and angry about divorce. They generally welcome the neutral and sympathetic help of a therapist. Older children are often deeply ashamed of their parents' divorce. They may have no one to talk to outside of the family; within the family, feelings may be so intense that safe discussion seems impossible.

The response of children to separation is often surprising to the parents. They have been so involved with their own miseries that there may have been little emotional energy to spare for their kids.

127

The parent may want to believe that the quality of life of the children will not change. It can be hard to imagine the fears and anger of the child faced with divorce. However, the child's feelings are real and often quite realistic. "Who will take care of me?" is the common concern. Many children blame themselves for the divorce. At a simple, common-sense, nonpsychiatric level, it is terribly important for parents to tell their children that the divorce is not their fault but that it is the responsibility of the parents themselves.

One pitfall for the practitioner is identifying with one of the parents in a separation. It can be hard to stay neutral. Most of us pediatricians have a closer relationship with the mothers in our practices than with the fathers, and we are most likely to hear the story of the split from them. The picture that is painted of the father can be pretty grim, but it is unlikely to be wholly accurate. On the other hand, a male physician may identify with the father, and of course, our own marital histories may make it difficult to stay objective. In any case, it is crucial to hear both sides of the story before giving advice. It is also worth talking to the kids; you may be able to help them through a very hard time. I have found that 30- to 45-minute appointments for the parents and perhaps as little as 15 minutes with the children are satisfactory.

One of the aspects about which you will be asked is child-sharing and custody, a rapidly changing area. A few decades ago, the typical pattern was for the children to stay with the mother; the father was limited to brief weekend and vacation contact with his children. In general, a mother had to be grossly incompetent to lose custody. All this has changed. Mothers as well as fathers work outside the home, and they are aware of the problems of single-parenting. Fathers increasingly want a substantial role in the upbringing of the children. The old pattern marginalized the father. He and his children could not develop a normal family pattern. The weekend daddy could have no real part in the everyday issues of raising children. He was limited to the role of the father who takes the kids to the movies or the zoo. For many men, paternal ties frayed, and they essentially disappeared from the lives of their own children.

Joint custody is the solution that has become popular. The idea is simple and attractive. Each parent provides a real home for the children, and the children shuttle back and forth on some kind of agreed rotation. (A much less common approach, sometimes termed "nesting," is for the children to stay in the family home while the parents come and go from their individual abodes; this is rarely attempted and even less commonly successful.) Joint custody clearly helps keep fathers involved; if you are spending several days every week with your children, it is harder to drop out. This solution maintains a reality-based parenting; each parent has the tasks of overseeing homework and household chores. It protects mothers from the pressures of working all day and single-parenting all evening. It also forces the parents to maintain a nonmarital but coparental relationship, which in the early years of a divorce can be excruciating. Eventually, most ex-marital partners learn to tolerate each other.

From the children's point of view, two houses sometimes mean no home. If one contemplates, from a parent's point of view, the "nesting" arrangement described earlier, the unsatisfactory nature of two houses becomes apparent. There is also the matter of the distance between the houses; two neighborhoods or two different cities mean disruption of the children's friendships. Where do the kids attend school, and who has to take them there? The question of separation is of particular importance for the infant and toddler; being away from either parent for several days can be exceedingly stressful. Usually this translates into being away from mother; she is likely to be the primary caregiver in the early years.

Even the most flexible arrangements can fail to meet everyone's needs, but on balance, some sort of shared custody makes the most sense most of the time.

Step-Parenting

What commonly follows divorce is the acquisition of a new marital partner, and thereby the creation of a step-parent. The usual first stage of this process is dating, which can be remarkably difficult for the adults and children alike. For the children of separated couples the appearance of dad's or mom's new date is awful confirmation that the separation is real and divorce imminent. It may also interrupt Oedipus- or Elektra-complex feelings; many a child has crept into the formerly marital bed when one partner has left it. When a more or less strange adult stays overnight in that bed for the first time, a certain amount of ill feeling can be expected.

If the new relationship becomes permanent, the step-parent is faced with the exceedingly complex task of developing a truly parental role in the family. This means becoming a rule-maker and rule-enforcer, taking over a fair share of the tasks of parenting, joining in the play and recreations of the family, making ties with the extended family—in short, acting like a mother or a father, rather than some sort of adult boarder. Sometimes real parental and filial love blossoms, which makes the role easier to fill; sometimes it doesn't happen. All this implies that becoming a step-parent requires an extraordinary degree of maturity and commitment. One is marrying a great deal more than a spouse. From the point of view of a mother or father, the new marriage requires a leap of faith that this new person will be a good parent for one's kids. Watching the process develop can be a prolonged ordeal; it does not always go smoothly.

Commonly, the new marital partners both bring children from a previous marriage into the new union. The problems increase exponentially, especially the problems of fairness, balancing all the claims for love, attention, and money among her kids and his kids. I list these issues not to suggest that there are solutions to them, but simply to indicate some areas in which problems will arise.

How to Be a Stepchild

If I had a chance to meet with the children in a newly forming stepfamily, these are some of the words of advice I would want to give them. The first rule, kids, is to stay out of the cross fire if you can. If you are already a child of divorce, you have had some practice with this. You may have learned to tell a parent you do not want to hear how awful your other parent was. When your parent and stepparent argue, suppress the natural tendency to kick someone in the shins; adults do not like being kicked. Second, recognize that this new adult has replaced the absent parent in your home but not in your heart. You do not have to reject the father who is no longer present in order to accept and even love the stepfather who is here now. Nor need you hate the stepfather in order to remain true to your dad. With luck, you can find what is strong and valuable to you in each relationship; do not expect this to happen quickly. Third, don't let anyone convince you that you have to love your stepsiblings; you may, in time, and they may love you. Initially, however, you may feel like you are in a litter in which the teats are outnumbered by the piglets.

The problem with all this wisdom is that it asks the child to hang in for the long haul. The formation of a well-functioning stepfamily is always slow, and rewards are not quickly forthcoming. However, that is the reality for everyone involved in a divorce, adults and children alike. The remarkable fact is that a substantial number of these new family structures work very well; this outcome requires enough time, lots of effort, and some exceptionally good luck.

❧ CHAPTER 12

Nutrition

We physicians have justly earned the reputation of nutritional nincompoops. Most medical schools provide little or no instruction in the field of nutrition. I presume that this situation exists largely because nutrition is mostly concerned with health, a concept difficult to define or study, and medical education is mostly concerned with disease, which is easier to define and more likely to be funded. Be that as it may, when I entered practice a number of mothers attempted to educate me about their True Beliefs Concerning Nutrition. I was given Adelle Davis's several books, as well as a variety of other True Believers' publications clarifying the mysteries of food and drink. Over the years the roles of vitamins, sugar, fats of all varieties, food additives, pesticides, yeast, simple and complex carbohydrates, fiber, excess protein, calcium, zinc, trace minerals, fluoride, and God only knows what else have been offered to the public by an amazingly diverse group of cranks and zealots and by an occasional real scientist. Sorting the wheat from the nutritional chaff is not always easy to do. The claims made are often exciting, sometimes upsetting, and rarely well-supported, but the subject is of sufficient importance that it merits our attention if not always our agreement.

Avoiding Allergy

It is a pity that a subject as important as food allergy is so hard to study. The results of about 70 years of investigation concerning the avoidance of food allergy during infancy seem quite unclear. A fair summary may be as follows.

First, if women with a personal history of major allergic disease could avoid large amounts of the most allergenic foods for all of pregnancy, the incidence of allergic disease in their children might diminish. Since this solution is impossible, it remains of academic interest only.

Second, early introduction of allergenic foods (cow's milk, egg white, orange, wheat, peanut, perhaps shellfish, fish, and corn) during infancy increases the incidence of infant eczema and possibly other allergic disease. It is not clear that protecting children from these allergens in infancy changes their later risk of allergic disease.

Growth and Nutritional Needs

Children's appetites are nearly unpredictably variable. A given child will eat vastly differing amounts from day to day for no discernible reason, and the differences among kids are amazing. About the only predictable pattern can be seen by looking at growth curves from birth to adolescence. The rapidly growing infant has a better appetite than the slower-growing toddler. Appetites during the years of early childhood tend to be modest. Most kids really eat only one or two good meals a day; they would generally rather snack. The growth curve of the adolescent girl is not as steep as her brother's curve; consequently, his adolescent growth spurt appetite will be much more impressive and expensive. During periods of slower growth and smaller appetites, most children narrow their range of preferred foods. Starches are the mainstay of children's diets during these periods especially. There is only a rough correlation between appetite and activity level, but generally children do eat more when they are most active. Eating is also a socially driven activity. You can get satiated chickens to eat more if you introduce some hungry chickens into their pen. A similar effect is seen with kids; they tend to eat more when they are with their friends.

Avoiding Nutritional Imbalance

Is it impious to discuss junk foods, juices, and milk in the same paragraph? Probably it is, but an old point is to be made again: nothing in excess. Fruit juices, the symbol of good health and proper parenting, are crummy foods. They provide sugar and water and that is about all, except for the vitamin C in orange juice and grapefruit juice and the vitamins C and A in tomato juice. Otherwise, they are the nutritional equivalents of ginger ale. Parents need to know that they rot teeth, limit appetite, and displace more useful foods. Milk is a good bit better, but because it is a low-iron food, an excess of milk in the early years will predictably lead to iron deficiency anemia. You see, nothing is sacred after all. What can be said about junk foods? Well, they actually have some redeeming qualities. There is vitamin C in french fries (13 mg in a regular order at McDonald's); there is a significant amount of calcium (581 mg) and protein (39 gm) in a 10-ounce serving of pizza. True, junk foods are generally very poor sources of minerals, vitamins, and fiber, and they tend to be major sources of salt, saturated fats, and sugar. Nevertheless, one must look at each junk food on its merits, insofar as it has any. An essential investment for the practitioner is Bowes and Church's *Food Values of Portions Commonly Used,* the standard source book of nutrition information, or the U.S. Department of Agriculture Agricultural Handbook No. 8, *Composition of Foods: Raw, Processed, Prepared* (available from the Superintendent of Documents, U.S. Government Printing Office, Washington, D.C. 20402, or the Department of Agriculture, Consumer Information Center, Pueblo, CO 81009). Browsing in either book is unexpectedly revealing. Perhaps the most important lesson for parents is that every morsel that passes their children's lips does not have to be maximally nourishing. Kids thrive on quite varied diets. Junk foods are like television; we are not going to keep our kids away from either, but we need to limit the ingestion of both.

Vitamin Supplements

Are there good reasons for adding supplemental vitamins to the diets of healthy American children? It is hard to find any data to support that practice. Vitamin A is easily available from milk; butter or margarine; cheese; eggs; carrots and other yellow, red, and green vegetables; and many fruits. The B vitamins are widely distributed in cereals, pasta and bread, nuts, peanuts, milk products, meats, and many vegetables. You are not going to come across pellagra or beriberi locally. Vitamin C is a little less ubiquitous. It is present in oranges, grapefruit, tomatoes, potatoes, leafy greens, cabbage family vegetables like broccoli, pineapple, berries, and melons. Vitamin D is in D-fortified milk (nearly all cow's milk sold in the United States is fortified), fatty fishes, and from sunshine. An eastern child who drank nonfortified milk directly from the family cow and who stayed inside the house during a long winter could manage to get rickets. There are actually some cases of rickets among inner-city, breast-fed black children. Their mothers are themselves vitamin D–deficient because their religion requires them to avoid exposure to the sun. In short, it is not easy to become vitamin D–deficient these days, but it can be done. Vitamin E is another easily available substance. The only cases of deficiency occurred a few years ago in premature babies fed an improperly processed commercial baby formula. Vitamin K is synthesized in the intestine; deficiency can occur in some malabsorption syndromes, and rarely in breast-fed infants during the first weeks of life.

So, who needs extra vitamins? Children with cystic fibrosis and other malabsorption diseases, food-allergic kids on restricted diets, and any children whose diets are grossly restricted by their own food preferences or other factors. Add to that list the kids whose parents are sure that extra vitamin C prevents colds; this is debatable but not terribly important. Surely the largest group needing extra vitamins are families in which parental anxiety is focused on food. If giving the kids an inexpensive, generic children's multivitamin takes some steam out of those households, it is not a bad investment.

What is the disadvantage of giving children extra vitamins? It is the metamessage that comes with the pill: "Good health comes out of a bottle." I think we should avoid this misteaching if we can.

Minerals

IRON

In earlier times, when our diet contained more whole grains and when our food was cooked in cast-iron pots, we Americans were less likely to become iron-deficient. Now, our diets can easily have marginal amounts of iron. We eat less meat and fewer eggs, both excellent iron sources. Many of us burn fewer calories at work and therefore eat less food, and many of us diet to lose weight. Any significant decrease in total intake will be likely to cut iron consumption to inadequate levels. This is a particularly common situation with teenage girls who are recurrently on diets, frequently less active than in earlier childhood, and losing blood with every menstrual period. Miss Average Teen can get pretty pale in a hurry. The other vulnerable group consists of babies and toddlers on fresh cow's milk, which provides practically no iron and can cause intestinal blood loss. If a child is thoroughly addicted to the bottle, the intake of iron-containing solids can be severely limited. However, for children in general, the iron fortification of cereals, breads, and other flour-based foods and the iron in peanut butter save the day.

If you have to treat an iron deficiency, keep in mind that the standard ferrous sulfate pills are highly toxic in an overdose, and they are easily mistaken for candy. Ferrous sulfate drops or syrups taste pretty bad; they also often cause temporary tooth discoloration, abdominal pain, and constipation. An expensive alternative that sometimes avoids these problems is a granular form (Feosol Capsules), which can be mixed into something like applesauce.

CALCIUM

Calcium is one mineral that may need to be added to quite a few childhood diets. The dietary sources are quite limited. Milk and milk products are certainly the best sources. Eggs and soy bean products have fair amounts, and there is some in broccoli and other leafy greens (perhaps not as well-absorbed) and in almonds. Calcium-fortified orange juice is another source. It is not a very long list. Supplementation by calcium carbonate or calcium phosphate is not difficult if the child can swallow a tablet; kids get quite resistant to chewing the flavored wafers (like Tums), which all eventually taste an awful lot like chalk. The calcium syrups are exceedingly expensive and disgustingly sweet.

FLUORIDE

The caries-controlling effect of fluoridated water is a true public health success story, and the leadership of the dental profession in fighting the battles for fluoridation has been exemplary. Fluoridated toothpaste, rinses, and local treatments have also helped, and caries has diminished even in areas with nonfluoridated water. It is certainly worthwhile to prescribe fluoride supplements for your patients whose drinking water is not fluoridated. If your patients come from several communities, you will need to call the various water companies serving them to find out whose water is fluoridated. Several words of caution are in order: (1) Very few families will continue to give fluoride supplements throughout the many years of tooth formation, from prenatal life until the midteens. Remind them! (2) An occasional family, usually led by a highly organized, compulsive professional, will never forget a dose! Their children will actually get more fluoride than they need, and their teeth, although as hard as rock, will show some white streaking on the anterior surfaces. These parents should be asked to give fluoride no more than five times a week and to skip the weekends. (3) The children of yuppies drink Perrier, which is not fluoridated. The children of health nuts drink exotically filtered waters or bottled spring water; these are all likely to be fluoride-deficient. Some children drink mostly soda pop and apple juice. Ask about these. (4) A wholly breast-fed baby probably gets a bit less fluoride than she needs. However, maternal fluoride levels have risen with the generally increased amount of fluoride in our diets, and some studies have shown an increase in the fluoride in mothers' milk. Furthermore, because most babies get some water in various ways, fluoride drops for these infants is needed only in nonfluoridated areas.

ZINC

Very rarely, an otherwise normal child manages to become zinc-deficient because of a bizarrely limited diet. This will lead to disorders of smell and taste, which cause anorexia and growth failure. The sequence is not easy to accomplish, because zinc is widely distributed in ordinary foods, but some kids can do it. Of course, zinc deficiency can also accompany protein-calorie malnutrition, acrodermatitis enteropathica, and a number of malabsorption states.

TRACE MINERALS

A few years ago, a considerable industry arose involving testing hair for mineral constituents, including a grand variety of trace elements. These hair analyses were then used as the basis for amazingly fanciful prescriptions designed to cure the deficiencies discovered. This particular form of technoquackery seems to have run its course.

Protein

A standard American diet supplies plenty of protein for standard American children. Remember that milk has about 1 gm protein per ounce, a slice of bread has 2 gm, a serving of dry cereal has 2 to 4 gm. The recommended level of 1 g/kg/d is easily met. A large proportion of our dietary protein is incomplete, lacking essential amino acids; this is especially true of the vegetable protein in cereals and legumes that make up a large part of the diet of children. Fortunately, a mixed diet of incomplete proteins works very well; rice protein plus bean protein is more complete and therefore more fully utilized than either alone. The same is true of wheat plus peanut; the peanut butter sandwich is truly the staff of life for the American child.

Carbohydrates

We certainly have strong feelings about foods. For years, carbohydrates were the least-honored constituent of our diets; people seemed to think of starches as fillers, pure and simple. Perhaps that is because they are low on the food chain and therefore less costly than proteins. In any case, things are changing. The contributions of complex carbohydrates to a balanced diet are now increasingly celebrated. Even diabetics are taught their virtues. Fortunately, starches are what children mostly want to eat; cereal, bread, pasta, rice, and potatoes. Of course, they also favor sugar, the simple carbohydrate, and, as every health "expert" knows, Sugar Kills. I regret to say that this lesson has been learned by every literate parent in my practice. The reality is less dramatic. It is true that sugar per se is an "empty-calorie" food, carrying no vitamins, protein, or minerals. A large sugar intake can certainly degrade the diet by displacing more complete foods. It is also true that a high-sugar diet is cariogenic. Can sugar make children hyperactive? When parents have reported this, I have had them test the theory by adding sugar to fruit juice or giving rock candy. On only one occasion did the parents see any relationship between extra sugar and a change in behavior. The usual report has been a rather disappointed "Nothing happened at all." Parents are often surprised to learn that white sugar, brown sugar, honey, molasses, and sugars from fruit all are essentially the same physiologically, since they all end up as glucose. In short, the case against sugar has been grossly overstated, and we all can relax.

Fats

The high priests of the diet-heart religion have bombarded us for quite some time with the message that Fat is Bad. As is often the case in theology, schisms have appeared. It is now rumored that mono-unsaturated fats like peanut oil and olive oil will be welcomed back into the fold of health-giving foods. There are even some whispers that not all polyunsaturated fats are created equal. For a period of fully half a year, it was accepted gospel that the n-3 fats found in fish oil were equivalent in value to the contents of the Holy Grail. This unhappily ethereal revelation has now been excluded from the canon. It now appears that lowering cholesterol levels with drug therapy actually seems to increase the risk of death from noncardiovascular causes. Whether diet therapy carries the same hazard is not clear. This leads to **Grossman's First Law of Medical Skepticism: Intensity of zealotry is directly proportional to muddiness of data.**

So, where does this leave our patients and their quest for The Right Fat? I think present information makes the following summary a reasonable starting place: (1) Moderate decreases in total fat intake are harmless and probably healthy. Because fat is a major source of calories, severe decreases in fat are usually unwise for growing children. (2) Fully saturated fats are the ones most likely to raise low-density lipoprotein cholesterol levels; a *modest* decrease in the amount of these fats by limiting fatty meat, butterfat, and other saturated cooking fats and oils like palm, cottonseed, and lard makes sense. (3) Monounsaturated olive and peanut oils and polyunsaturated oils are probably the most desirable from a cardiovascular point of view. (Remind parents that "old-fashioned" peanut butter, the kind that separates if not stirred, is preferable to the kind with hydrogenated oil.) (4) Since most human cholesterol is endogenously produced, limiting the intake of cholesterol per se is of less importance. In particular, avoiding the use of eggs, a highly nourishing food, is rarely indicated.

In short, switch to 2% milk, cut visible fat off meat, choose lower-fat meats like chicken and fish, and decrease the amount of sweets and desserts. These are mild diet changes that are likely to do no harm at all. Proposals to change the American diet in more radical ways should be approached with considerable caution. Well-meaning enthusiasm brought the starling to North America and the rabbit to Australia; the Aswan Dam did more for schistosomiasis than it did for Egypt; and DDT just about did in the pelican and the falcon. Experiments in nature can be hazardous.

Fiber

First let's dispose of the question of soluble fiber and blood lipids. It is claimed that oat bran and other sources of soluble fiber will decrease low-density lipoprotein cholesterol. Well maybe, but the quantities that seem to be required make this of academic interest only. How many oat bran muffins and bowls of oatmeal will any child willingly consume, and what difference would it make anyway? In contrast, indigestible fiber does seem to have significance for health, by virtue of its gastrointestinal effects. It passes into the large intestine, binds water, makes the stool bulkier and softer, and decreases intestinal transit time. Evidence is accumulating that a diet rich in fiber sources (whole grains, fruits, and vegetables) is associated with less gastrointestinal malignancy, diverticulitis, and possibly appendicitis. From the pediatric point of view, a high-fiber diet is the best single treatment for constipation. Unfortunately, most American kids eat refined grain products with little fiber. They also avoid most vegetables and frequently take their quota of fruit in fiber-poor juices. I am afraid that changing these patterns will require the efforts of a whole new group of zealots.

Vegetarian Diets

In my experience, families who have adopted a vegetarian diet are generally well-informed and well-fed. They usually know about the incomplete vegetable proteins. They all have studied Frances Moore Lappe's excellent book *Diet for a Small Planet* (Ballantine Books, New York, 1991). Most of them use milk products, making a good vegetarian diet a lot easier to achieve, and protecting them from vita-min B12 deficiency. They generally get adequate iron from cereals and legumes, although this can be a problem for adolescent girls and women, who lose iron with menstruation.

On the other hand, there is the mother who comes in with the frantic request, "What do I feed my teenager? She has decided to be a vegetarian!" This can be a setup for a great family struggle. Parents who are having any difficulty giving up control to an adolescent can become wonderfully embroiled in fights over what everyone is going to eat. The first necessity is educational; parents and children alike need to learn the basic facts of vegetarian nutrition. (Either *The New Laurel's Kitchen* by Laurel Robertson, Carol Flinders, and Bruce Rup-penthal, Ten Speed Press, Berkeley, CA, 1986, or Frances Lappe's book, already noted, is all they need.) The second issue is whether the family will change its diet; most families will not. This means parallel dinners, at least. Who has to do the extra work? If the new vegetarian wants to change her diet, she will generally be willing to plan her meals and cook them herself. If her more important agenda is fighting her folks and engendering extra guilt, the kitchen will be-come quite a battleground.

Additives, Coloring Agents, Salicylates, and Other Chemicals

This whole area of food additives is full of land mines. There is consid-erable scope for paranoia when one thinks about the terrible sub-stances being added to one's food. Even paranoids can have real ene-mies, and there are indeed examples of poisoning by food impurities. Between the real and the imagined dangers, it is not surprising that food additives are a touchy subject.

The additive that has received the most attention is monosodium glutamate (MSG), a flavor enhancer. It is widely believed to cause the "Chinese restaurant syndrome" of headache, breathing discomfort, and various other disorders of sensation. Evidence that such a reaction exists is surprisingly skimpy, but probably a very few people do have adverse responses to MSG (this substance is sometimes listed on food packages as "hydrolysed vegetable protein"). There is a similar dearth of evidence that food colors and salicylates in food cause trouble. The "Finegold diet," promulgated some years ago, attempted to cure hyperactivity and other behavior problems thought to be caused by these substances. The theory remains largely unsubstantiated, although I have seen a very few children who seemed to have behavioral changes after certain foods. More is said about this in the chapter on allergy.

The problem that currently causes the greatest concern to parents is pesticide and other chemical residues in foods. Are these carcinogens or mutagens? The size of the pertinent literature is matched by the intensity of feelings involved, which is a pretty good sign that not enough is known. I have been most impressed by the studies of Bruce Ames and Lois Gold.[1,2] They have concluded that the alleged risks have been greatly overemphasized by serious methodologic errors. I expect that we will continue to experience fiascos like the poisoned-cranberry scare of the 1960s, the nitrate scare of the 1970s, and the alar scare of a few years ago. All of these turned out to be embarrassingly overblown, but not before parental paranoia was turned up another notch.

[1] Ames BN, Magaw R, Gold L: Ranking Possible Carcinogenic Hazards. Science 1987; 236:271–280. Letters: 1987; 237, 235:1283–1284, 1399–1400; 1988; 238:1633–1634.
[2] Gold L et al: Rodent Carcinogens: Setting Priorities. Science 1992; 258:261–265.

✿ CHAPTER 13

Eating Problems and How to Induce Them

There can hardly be a more necessary biological function than the act of feeding one's children. The bond between infant and mother, in particular, is forged in the process of feeding. For many mothers, feeding becomes and remains the defining experience of being a parent. So we should not be surprised by the amount of emotional energy that parents invest in the questions of what and how much to feed their children. I think this is the context that must be kept in mind when we try to understand why a particular parent is acting in such a bizarre fashion about whether to give yellow or green vegetables first and other similarly earth-shaking issues. Aside from the biologic base, there are other factors that increase the tension surrounding feeding. The infant's growth and development are often perceived as validation of successful parenting; the big, plump infant proves the parents' success. No one ever coos over a baby, "Oh, what a darling, scrawny runt; you're certainly doing a great job with him."

As the child grows, sheer bulk loses its cachet; in fact, only large-boned and heavily muscled males are supposed to be really big after about age 1. The standards of the current social norms rapidly differentiate acceptable and nonacceptable shapes. In the United States today, the range of approved body styles is remarkably narrow, but the range of real anatomic variability in our species remains exceedingly wide. It is as if all dogs were supposed to be the size of cocker spaniels when in fact, dogs continued to come in sizes ranging from Great Dane to Chihuahua. The despair and concern among the owners of aberrant canines can be imagined. So it is with the parents of aberrant children. They want their kids to look like the standard

145

television family's child: moderately plump in babyhood, thereafter lean, muscular if male, lithe if female, above-average in height, tanned and blond if white, not too dark if black, preferably curly-haired, but not too curly. Unhappily, 95% of the time the kids diverge from this exemplary model; the parents may try to change reality by manipulating the diet. One of the most useful facts one can teach is that body size and shape are hardly at all amenable to these corrective efforts. The plump kid is probably going to be plump, pretty much along the lines of his plump parents; the skinny kid will not build massive muscles, no matter how much protein powder he consumes. Infinite perfectibility is a damaging myth.

This is particularly obvious in the current American view of obesity. It is worth recalling that overweight has not always been the object of so much disapproval. In societies of scarcity, to be fat means that one is rich and successful. The phrase "to carry weight" with ones peers implied the connection between power and bulk. Recall the pictures you have seen of Diamond Jim Brady or J. P. Morgan; they are not squash players. The favorite actresses of their day could be described as pleasingly plump or even generously endowed. Shakespeare's Julius Caesar said, "Let me have men about me that are fat," a viewpoint that would now get him in trouble with the cardiologists.

A reasonably balanced view of obesity needs to avoid the notion that being fat means that one is morally flabby. It seems clear that body shape is powerfully influenced by heredity. Twin studies and studies of adopted children confirm this. In the presence of adequate calories, children are going to grow pretty much as their DNA wants them to grow. Parents, diets, and weight reduction programs have no more than a peripheral effect. This somewhat uncomfortable but inexorable fact leads directly to **Grossman's First Law of Weight Control: If you can't do anything useful, don't do anything at all.** The reason behind this piece of therapeutic nihilism is simple. When you prescribe a course of weight reduction or diet change that is going to fail, you injure the child. The sequence is nearly invariable: (1) Weight is lost. (2) Everyone feels triumphant and wonderful. (3) Weight is regained, and the growth chart is right back at 2½ standard deviations above the mean, just like it was 6 months ago before the diet. (4) Everyone feels awful and defeated. The child's view of himself as a moral and physical slob with no will power at all is confirmed.

I think the practitioner's best role in weight control should be in teaching that people come in all shapes and sizes and that not much can be done about it. Furthermore, from the perspective of physical health, moderate overweight is of little or no importance. Help the child to accept the fact that she is curvier than the fashion models and that the fault lies in the societal norms. Add to this a modest amount of information about the virtues of physical activity and the caloric content of foods, and you have given her about all that medical science can offer. Neither you nor your patient will be satisfied, but you will at least have spoken up for sanity and perhaps helped to protect the child from the damaging social pressure to be slim.

Of course, skinny kids have social pressures too, but theirs seem much milder. The very slender boy will yearn for more muscle from middle childhood onward. He may need to hear that special diets are quite useless and weight-training exercises not much better. Slenderness in girls is only rarely perceived as a problem in childhood, although these children may want to be less linear once adolescence arrives.

Back in the 1930s the Duchess of Windsor said, "You can never be too rich or too thin." This nonsense qualifies her as the patron saint of the current epidemic of anorexia nervosa and bulimia. The early studies of anorexic youngsters focused on specific family patterns. These girls (rarely boys) came from smart, demanding, and controlling parents more often than not. The girl's struggle to separate from her mother and to accept her own developing sexuality appeared to be central issues in the genesis of the disorder. Many of these patients were profoundly emotionally disturbed. Even with skillful and prolonged treatment, the eventual outcome was often not wholly satisfactory. Eating problems often persisted for decades.

These cases of classic anorexia were rarities. In our pediatric group practice, we might see one every few years, but in the last decade, anorexia and bulimia have become absolutely commonplace. At any time in our practices now there will be several anorexics and probably even more bulimics. A few of the anorexics are severely disturbed girls with life-threatening disease, but most of them seem rather different. They may have similar psychodynamic problems, but at a less severe level. These girls do not seem to have as much distortion of their body images. Insight into the problems comes more easily, and they seem to recover more rapidly and more completely. It is my sense that they are basically sturdier people, less in the grip of family struggle than the classic anorexics, but perhaps more influenced by social pressures to be slim.

The management of these conditions starts with a sharp eye and an accurate scale. Unexplained weight loss requires your interest and attention. It may take some time before you can convince yourself and the family that a significant problem exists. You may find that the patient resists the diagnosis, and you may be sure that she will resist the therapy. These kids need a skillful psychotherapist, preferably one who will work with the family as well as the patient herself. Some therapists work with groups of anorexics or bulimics, which is a good measure of how common these conditions have become. Recently, there is interest in the use of antidepressants, especially for bulimics. The pediatric management is straightforward. I explain the physical risks of starvation and outline the measures to avoid it, including weekly office visits to monitor weight, blood pressure, and pulse and to watch for the usual changes in hair and skin. Constipation and amenorrhea are nearly always present. The child needs to know something about minimal dietary necessities; it is usually a good idea to prescribe multivitamins, calcium, and iron. I urge the parents to stop telling the child how much and what to eat; feeding is a function that must be taken over by the girl herself. This is because increasing control of her life is a necessary part of her recovery; the struggle over food is really a symbol of the more general issues of maturing and individuating.

A lowest allowable weight is defined, and I explain that the girl will be hospitalized if her weight falls below that point. Sometimes I allow a few days to regain an acceptable weight. The family and the girl are told that if hospital care is needed, a measured diet will be offered. If it is not taken, the needed nourishment will be given by nasogastric tube. Discharge from the hospital will be possible only when a new, higher target weight is reached. During the most acute phase of anorexia, the behavior of some of the girls reminds me of the behavior of drug addicts. They lie blandly about their eating habits, drink massive amounts of water, or hide sacks full of sand inside their underwear just before a weigh-in visit, and they generally drive their parents to distraction. The pressure on these families is intense and prolonged. The parents are faced with a child's suicidal rebellion. They are frantic with worry for months, and they also are furious about the child's dangerous behavior. Usually they blame themselves for the illness. They need continued support from the pediatrician, and they need a good psychotherapist for themselves. In some tough cases, the pediatrician may feel the need for a little personal psychotherapy as well.

The socially aware reader will note that I have not mentioned the most common feeding problem faced by the children of the world: not enough to eat. Even in the United States today, one out of three children grows up in a home in poverty, and poverty means hunger. Glib advice falls silent in the face of that painful reality.

❦ CHAPTER 14

Constipation

Because I was raised as a Freudian, my early understanding of constipation was psychological; there were all those anal-retentive people who could presumably be analyzed into comfortable regularity. Well, perhaps there are some such aspects to the problem, but at least in pediatric practice, genetics, diet, and activity patterns seem to be determining factors.

Genetics to begin with: there really are constipated families. Whether these people have unresponsive bowels or superefficient water recycling mechanisms I don't know, but the mother who reports constipation in her infant and comments that half the adults in her family need laxatives has my full attention. These children often have a recurrent pattern of constipation that requires careful dietary manipulation for years.

Diet is certainly the most important factor in bowel function. It is usually said that breast-fed babies are never constipated, and like so much that is "usually said," this is nearly true. The once-every-feeding, loose-to-watery stools of the nursing infant commonly diminish in frequency during the first few months, sometimes to a single stool every few days. The record in my practice is one stool per 2 weeks. These infrequent stools are soft and painless when they are passed; however, some babies will be fretful for as much as a day prior to producing a generous stool. It may be worth giving them a feeding of sugar water or molasses water to stimulate a stool. Adding sugar or molasses to the formula is also useful in bottle-fed babies, who certainly can get constipated; molasses is more effective but messier. One half to 1 teaspoon of either can be added to as many bottles a day as required; the dose is titrated against the results. Malt soup extract is a more expensive alternative. Constipation may actually be due to food allergy; you may need to change from a cow's milk formula to soy or Nutramigen.

When constipation is present in infancy, one obviously has to consider anatomic abnormalities, including Hirschsprung's disease and rectal or anal malformations. Recently, the claim has been advanced that a minimal anterior displacement of the anus is a common cause of constipation; I keep looking for this problem but so far without success.

When solid foods are introduced, constipation problems increase; this is usually caused by an excess of baby cereal. One should give less cereal and add fruits; peaches and plums give better results than do applesauce or bananas. The worst transition is to fresh milk; to avoid constipation at weaning from formula or breast, fresh cow's milk should be added a little at a time over a few weeks.

After infancy, the important dietary factor in constipation is lack of fiber. Unfortunately, the American child's diet of peanut butter on white bread, pizza, Frosted Flakes, sweets, Coke, and apple juice doesn't provide much indigestible roughage. It is quite a task to help families change to a diet with more whole grain breads and cereals, fresh fruit, and water; less juice and soda pop; and fewer concentrated sweets. More vegetables would also be a help, but that option is quite out of reach.

Lack of water seems to be a problem for a few children; it should not be solved by offering juice, because the extra calories may replace solid foods that could have provided fiber as well.

Nondietary factors include providing enough time for the child to recognize the urge to stool and do something about it; this is no mean feat on busy school-day mornings. The small child may also need some place to plant his feet if there is any need to strain at stool; this is one reason potty chairs on the floor are better than the ones that perch on the regular toilet seat. During the period when toilet training is under way, the bowel movement may become the center of a vigorous power struggle between parents and child. Refusing to use the potty and fearing disapproval for using the diaper may set up a considerable case of constipation. Unfortunately, the current American custom of bowel training at 2 to 2½ years coincides with the period of the child's maximum independence needs. It is a good trick to convince a wily and surly kid that using the toilet is somehow in his best interests and is not just a present to his parents. Rewards help.

The most difficult problems arise when a child has had a painful, hard stool and fears the next bowel movement. This often starts the common pattern of withholding stool and getting more and more obstipated. Mineral oil is usually sufficient to soften and lubricate the stool, but sometimes enemas or even digital disimpaction is needed. Mineral oil is best given shaken with a little orange juice; one should start with ½ tablespoon twice a day and increase slowly until the stools are so runny that the child can't withhold. The mineral oil is slowly decreased over several weeks, during which time one hopes that the child will decide that bowel movements are acceptable. An expensive alternative to mineral oil is lactulose, a nonabsorbable sugar that increases stool water content. Sometimes it works fairly well. Docusate sodium is a mildly effective lubricant-cathartic; its popularity with pediatricians is largely due to its ease of administration. It does not suffice in the treatment of withholding. Stimulant laxatives should be avoided because they can cause severe cramps, may fail to soften the stools adequately, and may be habituating. Obviously, attention must also be paid to the antecedents of the withholding, or the cycle may just repeat itself.

Brown clay play is often a useful adjunct with small kids; a parent sits down with the child, a doll or two, a potty chair, and some soft brown clay. If one says, "Let's play that the doll doesn't want to use the potty," most children enter into a useful and therapeutic interaction. A few brief play periods like this may be needed.

Constipation may also be caused by illness, bed rest, or drugs; it is not always preventable, but timely use of milk of magnesia, bisacodyl, or mineral oil will cure it.

Encopresis may result from a number of causes. Sometimes complete toilet training seems not to be accomplished for years, and a little soiling comes to be accepted by child and family as just the way things are. More often soiling begins when a child who has previously mastered toileting becomes constipated, withholds stool, and overflows. Not infrequently, encopresis is part of a major problem in child-family interaction. The pediatrician can approach this symptom warily, hoping that clearly stated parental expectations plus proper medical and dietary management will suffice. If this fails, counseling or formal psychotherapy is the next step.

❧ CHAPTER 15

Enuresis

If you try to teach 5-year-old children to read, a large number of them will fail to master the task, and you will be well on the way to creating a cadre of children with reading problems. If you wait until the children reach age 6 or 7 before making this attempt, the proportion of failures will be much smaller, because maturation of the necessary neural networks will have taken place; many fewer of these children will be defined as having reading problems. Exactly the same situation is true for bed-wetters. If you provide children with big enough diapers for a long enough time and keep adult expectations sufficiently relaxed, many fewer children will be defined as enuretic. In short, primary nocturnal enuresis is not a disease; it is one stage in a developmental process.

Like all biologic functions, the acquisition of control over urination during sleep is subject to immense variability. There are a few children of age 18 or 20 months who awaken dry in the morning and toddle off to the potty. In contrast, there are 7- or 8-year-olds who sleep peacefully through the night in a bed awash with the results of multiple micturitions. Heredity plays a role here; parents often relate an identical personal history of prolonged bedwetting. These children are also usually described as wonderfully deep sleepers: "You couldn't wake him with a cannon." A quite different matter is secondary enuresis, the resumption of bed-wetting by the child who had once achieved night dryness. These children may have a variety of systemic illnesses, urinary tract infection, urethral or vaginal irritation, pinworms, or diabetes. Even more likely, they may be reacting to psychological stress; if the physical exam, urinalysis, and urine culture are all negative, that's where the money is.

Daytime enuresis is more complicated. Once again, expectations are a factor. Many normal 3- and 4-year-olds still wet themselves fairly regularly during the day, but by 6 or 7 years of age, more than an occasional dribble deserves some attention. Some of these children show other signs of neurologic or developmental delay. A very few prove to have genitourinary anomalies or infection. Some are said to have a learned dysfunction of urination, although I have some doubts about this. Most of these kids seem to me to be peeing on their parents; the wet pants are a part of a larger family struggle.

Management of primary enuresis starts with prevention. Set parental expectations at a realistically low level. About 50% of children will be dry at night by 3 years of age, the girls tending to develop bladder control earlier than the boys. If you know that a parent or a sibling was a bed-wetter, remind the family that this pattern can be expected to repeat itself. Try to define this as a problem for the bed rather than for the child. The availability of large diapers or "pull-ups" is a help. If this is not acceptable, the child's bed can be protected by a large rubber-backed cotton felt pad. As the child gets older, he can take responsibility for airing his bed every morning, changing it when necessary, and helping with the family laundry. This is a nonpunitive but precise message to him that a dry bed is a valuable goal. Eventually, family and social pressure will make more active measures advisable. Behavior modification techniques such as rewards for dry nights are sometimes remarkably effective. A prominently displayed star chart with a star for each dry night and a specific reward for a defined number of stars is the usual tactic. The interesting feature of this method is that it can be abandoned once continence is achieved, with only a small likelihood of relapse. Real learning seems to take place.

If the star chart fails, alarm devices are the next step. These consist of moisture detectors worn in the child's underpants with a wire connected to a buzzer near the child's ear. (The earlier models, which had a moisture detecting pad placed under the bed sheet, were much less reliable.) When the child begins to urinate, the alarm sounds, awakening him and usually his parents. He is then supposed to go to the toilet to finish urinating. The theory is that he will awaken sooner and sooner, eventually somehow learning to respond to the preceding neural stimulus of a full bladder. Presumably he will either inhibit the impulse to void or he will awaken and trudge to the toilet instead. The theory carries little conviction, but the practice often works. Problems arise when the child manages to stay asleep despite the noise of the alarm; parents and siblings are often more easily aroused than the patient. An extra loud alarm is available with some of these gadgets; this is by no means uniformly successful, and it may just make the rest of the family even angrier. Alarm devices are useless if the child is not motivated to become dry. It is also a waste of time to use them before age 5 or 6 years at the earliest.

The last resort is medication. Imipramine decreases or stops bed-wetting for at least half of enuretic children, but relapses are disappointingly common. Toxicity is dose-related and can be serious; don't push past the recommended level. Sometimes the combination of imipramine plus an alarm device is helpful. One can also use imipramine for a few days or weeks to help a child control bed-wetting during a vacation or at summer camp, with the expectation that relapse will occur later. Desmopressin has recently been tried on the basis of the theory that these kids just don't concentrate their urine at night in the usual fashion. Unfortunately, relapse after the conclusion of therapy is the rule, and the cost is astronomical.

Keep in mind the damp, unhappy reality that some kids take forever to sleep dry. It can be a long wait until night-time continence is finally established in the teens, but it does eventually happen.

❧ CHAPTER 16

Developmental Orthopedics

My old chief Ed Shaw used to say that a practicing pediatrician needed to know three kinds of surgeons: one who always wanted to operate, one who never wanted to operate, and one who knew how to think. I am reminded of this cynical advice in regard to the treatment of the minor positional deformities of the lower extremities in newborns. If your local orthopedic surgeon belongs in the first category of therapeutic enthusiasts, you and your patients are in for a lot of trouble. Fortunately, observation has largely replaced intervention, as practitioners have noted that most of these conditions spontaneously resolve over time. The days when casts, splints, and corrective shoes were *de rigueur* have passed.

When you examine a newborn and discover turned-in feet or twisted tibias and the like, you are generally witnessing the result of a tight fit in the uterus. During the last months, the fetus has adopted a position of comfort, and this has allowed bones and soft tissues to become surprisingly asymmetrical. The entire lower extremity can be affected. In most but not all cases, release from the prison of the womb plus the normal processes of growth will correct the initial deformity. A caveat must be noted: some familial deformities can look just like these transient positional conditions. If mom or dad has bowed legs or other abnormalities of the extremities, baby may have the same.

Anteversion of the Hips

Anteversion of the hips, one of the less common of these intrauterine position problems, is also the least likely to resolve completely. In this condition, the femurs are twisted medially, the femoral neck pointing in a more anterior direction than normal. The lower extremities thus rotate toward the midline; the knees point medially when the child lies supine. This may become more obvious as the child grows. It can be confused with tibial torsion, because both conditions turn the feet medially. However, unlike tibial torsion, anteversion of the hips may persist. Twister devices and Denis Browne splints are equally useless. This is an essentially harmless anatomic variant, which must be recognized and ignored.

Tibial Torsion

Tibial torsion is a different matter. Here the tibia has more than the usual mild bowing seen in most babies. The medial twist of the tibia turns the ankle and foot inward into a striking and sometimes asymmetrical pigeon-toe. This used to stimulate a frenzy of treatment. The minimum effort was the application of Denis Browne splints attached to firm, high-topped, orthopedic shoes. The shoes were rotated outward to put a torque on the tibia. This many-months-long ordeal eventuated in straighter tibias, but the effects on the knees were not always good. Treatment finally moved toward sanity when the Denver Growth Study showed that tibial torsion disappeared spontaneously in nearly all instances. At present, a reasonable approach is watchful waiting, or what the English clinicians used to call "masterful inactivity." Over a period of 3 or 4 years, twisted tibias grow into a straighter shape; it is a slow process. A remarkably severe case or one with striking asymmetry between the two sides might rarely lead one to consider Denis Browne splints, but they should be avoided, if possible.

Calcaneovalgus Deformity

A common and even less important deformity is the foot bent back against the front of the skin, the calcaneovalgus deformity. These are quite flexible feet and ankles and are easily placed in a normal position. In some instances there is an associated forefoot valgus; that is, the forefoot is bent laterally while the entire foot is lying in a strongly dorsiflexed position. This deformity self-corrects within months. Make sure that lower extremity reflexes and muscle activity are normal to avoid confusion with neuromuscular disorders.

Metatarsus Varus

Deviation of the forefoot toward the midline is termed metatarsus varus or metatarsus adductus. In this common condition, the soft tissues of the inner edge of the foot are contracted, but the foot can be pulled rather easily into a neutral position. Left alone, metatarsus varus may improve to a degree, but complete resolution cannot be counted on. This is one positional deformity that requires treatment. Stretching exercises should be instituted in very early infancy. The caretaker holds the hindfoot firmly in one hand and with the other hand bends the forefoot laterally. The proximal portion of the fingers next to the lateral edge of the baby's foot act as a fulcrum for the bending motion. The stretched position is held for several seconds and then relaxed. The stretching is repeated over a 2-minute period; the force exerted is guided by the baby's tolerance. Try to pull the forefoot past neutral into a valgus position; after the first few days of stretching, this should be accomplished with ease. At least two or three sessions a day are needed to make reasonable progress, and many months will be required to bring the feet into a truly neutral position. These feet tend to slip back to a varus deformity if stretching is abandoned too early. Rarely, an out-flared stiff shoe or orthopedic boot can be used for follow-up control. At times, stretching does not succeed, generally because neither babies nor parents enjoy the process. If you cannot convince the family to work harder at this routine, the baby will need serial casting by an orthopedist.

Congenital Dislocation of the Hip

Congenital dislocation of the hip is another condition in which intra-uterine position and crowding play a part, although gender and heredity may be more important factors. For the purposes of this discussion, two points need to be noted. Neither dislocation nor subluxation of the hip is necessarily present at birth; repeated, gentle examinations of the hips should be done, at least until the child is walking normally. When a hip is noted to be unstable but not frankly dislocated at birth, instant treatment is not necessary. One can obtain a sonogram, and then watch and wait. A lot of these babies' hips tighten up nicely with no help at all.

Flexible Flatfoot

After infancy, other developmental foot problems can make an appearance. One of the most common is flexible flatfoot. Of course, the pudgy foot of the baby with its pad of fat obscuring the arch looks flat. As a more mature shape evolves, true flatfoot is often seen. When the foot is examined in the absence of weight-bearing, the longitudinal arch is usually present, although rather shallow. Viewed from the rear of the standing child, the pronation is obvious; the arch collapses, the heel slants inward and the Achilles tendon insertion looks concave. These kids often have generally loose ligaments and more than usual flexibility of all their joints. In early and middle childhood, flatfoot is typically asymptomatic, and with time most children's feet improve. A few children remain flat-footed into adolescence, but only rarely does this condition become the source of discomfort. In these instances, firm arch supports are a real help; sometimes plastic orthotics prescribed by a podiatrist are necessary.

Bunions

A less common condition is hallux valgus and the development of bunions. This condition seems to depend on two factors. First, there is probably an inherited medial (varus) deviation of the first metatarsal, which pushes the great toe medially as well. Second, there is the countervailing force of the shoe, pushing the distal portion of the great toe in the opposite direction. The result is an increasing prominence and angulation of the first metatarsophalangeal joint, a bunion, which is painfully constrained by the medial border of the shoe. This condition is much more common in girls and women, probably because the design of their shoes from infancy onward is so ridiculously unanatomic. The pointed-toe shoe should be avoided whenever possible.

"Ingrown Toenails"

The shoe industry is also partially responsible for the condition misnamed "ingrown toenails." This tends to be an affliction of big adolescent males with wide forefeet. Even the currently popular soft footwear of the young is designed with inadequate toe room, both vertically and horizontally. At every step, the toes are constricted and formed into a sort of digital wedge pushing into the tip of the shoe. The adolescent foot grows with astounding speed, and shoes are often worn for months after the available toe space has been used. This problem tends to be obscured by the design of the shoe, which retains some apparent space where it is not useful, at the tip of the shoe distal to the third toe. The effect of this wedging is to push the great toe toward the second toe, which cannot move out of the way. The soft tissue of the inner aspect of the great toe is trapped between the great toenail and the second toe. It responds by becoming swollen and it overgrows the inner edge of the great toenail. If this problem is ignored for a long enough time, a red, tender, purulent mass develops.

Treatment is slow and relapses are common, because the feet keep growing and the shoes don't fit. The following approach works fairly well.

1. Get the child out of the offending shoes. If possible, the child should wear sandals, go barefoot, or wear a shoe with the toe cut away until healing has occurred.

2. Soak the foot for 10 to 15 minutes at least two times a day in hot, soapy water.

3. After the soak, express any pus from around the nail, and push the soft tissues laterally with a cotton swab.

4. If the infected area is draining, apply a blob of antibiotic ointment covered by a small bandage.

5. Let the great toenail grow out; when it needs trimming, cut it straight across rather than convex. (Sometimes a spicule of

nail is present at the lateral border; if so, the practitioner will need to trim it off. This hurts.)

6. A systemic antibiotic like amoxicillin-clavulanate or a cephalosporin may be needed for 1 or 2 weeks.

7. In rare instances, it is necessary to anesthetize the toe with a digital block and to remove about one-third of the nail from the border next to the second toe. This is easily done by using a heavy clamp to grasp the nail and heavy straight scissors to cut the nail all the way down to the base. The nail will slowly grow back to its usual shape, giving plenty of time for healing to occur.

8. The last resort, when recurrences continue, is ablation of part of the nail matrix so that the nail is made permanently narrower.

9. Prevention consists of warning kids with big, wide feet that cramped toes cause a lot of trouble. They need the bluntest, widest-toed shoes they can find.

Fitting Children's Shoes

As I hope has been made clear, properly fitted shoes can go a long way toward preventing certain foot problems. Unfortunately, parents often have the notion that fitting a shoe is an esoteric and difficult art, best left to its practitioners in shoe stores. This is nonsense. Parents need to understand the following.

1. Shoes are basically protective garments. They should keep feet comfortable, somewhat cushioned from hard surfaces, dry during wet weather, and protected from a variety of road hazards like broken glass and dog feces. With the rare exception of orthopedic shoes for true deformities, shoes do not aid in the development of normal feet. The longer babies and children can go barefoot, the better.

2. What Jefferson said about government can be said about shoes: the least shoe possible is best. Heavy, stiff, high-topped

shoes are too hot, too hard to put on, too expensive, and too hard to fit accurately. Soft sandals and moccasins are best for babies and toddlers.

3. Feet grow. The child being fitted should stand up in the new shoes. There should be at least ½ inch of space distal to the great toe, with plenty of room vertically and horizontally. A boxy toe is best. There must also be room for growth across the ball of the foot; one should be able to pinch up loose fabric or leather at the widest part of the forefoot. The ball of the foot should be at the widest part of the shoe.

4. Shoes are expensive; hand-me-downs are perfectly acceptable if they fit and if the previous wearer did not grossly distort the shape of the shoes.

5. Shoes should no longer be worn when the available toe and forefoot room has been outgrown. This often means new shoes of a larger size are needed every month or so during the adolescent growth spurt.

CHAPTER 17

The Skin: General Care and Common Problems

Children's skin is second only to the respiratory tract in frequency as the site of medical problems. Because the patterns of difficulty are age-dependent, this discussion proceeds from infancy to adolescence.

❧ INFANT SKIN

The skin of newborn babies is a fairly effective and reasonably healthy material, if we would only leave it alone. Unfortunately, patterns of skin care in infancy tend to be intrusive and vigorous, and even the best-designed integument can get into trouble. The first mistake we make is the excessively thorough bath soon after birth. The lubricating vernix is scrubbed away, and the baby's skin responds by becoming dry and cracked. By the second day one often sees a little bleeding, especially at the wrists and ankles. This should be a hint that we are doing something wrong, but the routines of hospital nurseries seem to be immune to rationality. Luckily, infants heal quickly if the family can be persuaded to limit further ablutions. Most babies do very nicely with a bath every few days plus an occasional rinse of the diaper area. Any mild soap will suffice; there is absolutely no reason to believe that special soaps are useful. It is often suggested that infants should be sponge-bathed, rather than be immersed in water, until the umbilicus has healed; great efforts are expended to keep the cord stump dry. This notion would be hilarious if it were not so much trouble. The umbilical cord has been soaking in fluid for all of fetal life. How continued intermittent moisture could be dangerous is a considerable mystery. Washing the baby's face and hair is best done with a "baby" shampoo to avoid eye irritation. The significant difference between these products and standard shampoos is the presence of an amphoteric buffering agent. The only other rules for the routine care of infant skin are to avoid overheating the baby with excessive clothing and overheated rooms and to avoid cosmetics like baby oil, powder, and lotion.

Baby Acne

Within the first weeks of life, a substantial number of infants develop tiny red or white pimples and pustules, first appearing on the scalp and forehead, then extending down the face and onto the shoulders. This is most commonly seen in babies with oily skin and often is accompanied by the greasy scale of seborrhea. Left alone, baby acne subsides over a few more weeks. It tends to flare temporarily when the baby is overheated. Gentle washing seems mildly helpful. In extreme cases, when the parents are terminally upset by the baby's prematurely adolescent appearance, one can calm down both skin and family with ½% hydrocortisone cream used b.i.d.

Seborrhea

Sometimes baby acne segues into the more chronic problem of infant seborrhea. This disorder of scaling has several presentations. The most common is cradle cap, the yellow-brown scaly or greasy material that clings to the infant's scalp. You will notice that cradle cap is heaviest over the fontanels, where the parents are afraid to scrub vigorously. This is one condition for which frequent and muscular washing is often all that is needed. Rarely one may need to use a sulfur and salicylic acid shampoo; even less often, a liquid corticosteroid (halcinonide or fluocinolone) may be used very briefly and sparingly. More widespread forms of seborrhea show up as scale, which looks like finely crushed potato chips clinging to the eyebrows and cheeks. This can become generalized over the trunk, and it is not always possible to differentiate it from infant eczema. Unlike eczema, seborrhea is usually not pruritic; it often has an accompanying red, moist intertrigo of the axillae, neck, and inguinal creases. With eczema, in contrast, the antecubital and knee creases tend to be red, and there is often some central pallor in the crease. I think some children have both, a seborrheic eczema that is widespread and persistent; these cases are hard to control. In general, seborrhea is best dealt with by frequent bathing to remove the scale. Medicated soaps and cleansers with sulfur or salicylic acid can be used; tar-containing cleansers are also effective, but most parents object to having their infants smell like a newly paved street. Hydrocortisone creams of ½% or 1% are safe and effective. Secondary infection with *Staphylococcus* or yeast may require treatment as well. The use of a barrier cream containing silicone can help to protect the face and neck from irritation by saliva and food.

Eczema

The typical appearance of eczema in early infancy is the red-cheeked baby with red antecubital spaces, rubbing her face back and forth to relieve the itching. The rash often spreads to the trunk and inguinal creases; on the extremities eczema is most concentrated on the wrists, knee creases, and ankles. In later infancy, the truncal rash may be patchy and coinlike (nummular). When eczema is severe and persistent, the most easily scratched lesions become thickened. Secondary infection with *Staphylococcus* is exceedingly common.

A predominant factor in the development of infant eczema is food allergy. If the mothers in your practice breast-feed and keep fresh cow's milk, orange juice, egg white, and wheat out of the babies' diets, you will see a lot less infant eczema. In later infancy, other foods are possible culprits, in particular, peanut butter, corn, soy, fish, and shellfish. Factors other than food allergy are increasingly important at older ages: contactants, either as allergens or as irritants, and a tendency toward dry skin. Etiology changing with age is one reason for the disagreements about the cause of eczema. Dermatologists rarely have the opportunity to see the classic food-triggered eczema of infancy. They tend to treat eczema with little regard to allergic factors and therefore miss the possibility of effecting a prompt cure by dietary changes.

Some rules governing successful management of eczema are independent of the etiology. In general, eczematous skin is dry, and anything making it drier will usually make it worse. Bathing removes the skin oils, which tend to maintain moisture. Soap is the worst offender, but even water alone can be damaging. Bathing should be minimized; baths should be brief and soapless, if possible. If some kind of cleanser is needed, one should use a mild soap like Dove or a soapless lotion like Cetaphil. Immediately after a bath, while the skin is hydrated, an emollient cream can be used to trap some of this water within the skin. Eucerin, Cetaphil, Keri Lotion, Nivea cream, and many other similar products are available. For really mild cases of eczema, emollients used twice a day may be sufficient. The mainstay of topical medication is the old faithful 1% hydrocortisone cream. It works, it has very little systemic effect, it rarely stings, and it is wonderfully inexpensive. A small application two or three times a day will control the majority of eczemas. Unlike the more powerful topical steroids, it can be used (but sparingly) on the face and in the diaper area. The 1% hydrocortisone fails when used on old, lichenified lesions. These are hard to handle, even with the strongest steroids; use a class 2 steroid like halcinonide or betamethasone diproprionate in an ointment rather than in a cream or lotion base. You may find that the expensive, branded products are best; some generic topical steroids don't seem to be properly formulated.

The dietary approach to treatment for eczema is easy if the baby has not yet started solid foods. Eczema due to food allergy in a wholly breast-fed infant is truly a great rarity. If you come across such a case, a rational approach would be a hypoallergenic diet for the mother. At a minimum, this would mean excluding milk, milk products, eggs, wheat, corn, soy, oranges, peanuts, fish, and shellfish from her diet for a 2- to 3-week trial. If the eczema starts to subside, foods are reintroduced, one at a time, every 3 to 5 days, and the effect observed. If the baby is formula-fed, one should switch to a casein hydrolysate like Nutramigen. If the taste and expense of Nutramigen are problems, a soy formula could be tried, but many atopic infants do not tolerate soy any better than cow's milk. During diet trials, one may be tempted to start topical treatment as well. If at all possible, one should resist the urge; it will complicate subsequent efforts to understand what happened and why.

The older infant who develops eczema after solid foods have been introduced poses a harder problem. Of course, the rash may have flared up within a few days after a new food was started. If so, stop the new food and observe. If there is no obvious candidate for exclusion, stop all the allergenic foods already mentioned or, if necessary, all solids of any kind. If baby or parents demand solids, the following foods are least likely to be allergens: lamb, white potato, sweet potato, spinach, carrot, pear, peach, apricot, plum, and rice (including rice crackers and baby rice cereal). A period of 2 to 3 weeks on an elimination diet usually leads to improvement. The parents must be warned to study labels. Foods fortified with vitamins and minerals pose no problem, but additions of flour, starches, sweeteners, and flavorings should be avoided.

Elimination diets are difficult to manage. There is always an older sibling or a grandmother giving the baby an unauthorized treat, or an unexpected additive in an otherwise innocent jar of baby food. Furthermore, eczema waxes and wanes without obvious cause. You may have to remove and return a food from the diet on more than one occasion to convince yourself of its effect. Practitioners and families can get very tired of diet manipulation, but it works.

Diaper Rashes

Note the plural. "Diaper rash" is a wastebasket diagnosis and like all wastebaskets, has a variety of contents. What these rashes have in common is occurrence in an area of skin subject to multiple indignities including immersion in urine and stool, abrasion from diapers, increased heat due to occlusive coverings, and nearly constant moisture. This last factor explains why the diaper area is so unlikely to be involved in infant eczema; the hydration reverses the skin dryness that is a major part of eczema.

Most diaper area rashes are transient and unimportant contact irritations set off by neglect of sufficiently frequent diaper changing or by careless hygiene or excessively tight diapers. The currently popular paper diapers with elastic edges often cause linear patches of skin redness, especially if the baby is too plump or too muscular for an easy fit. Rarely, the offending contactant is a urinary constituent; I have seen an occasional case due to sensitivity to orange juice. Treatment consists of correcting the apparent cause, exposing the diaper area to air and a little sun, if available, and protecting the skin with a barrier ointment. All the various zinc oxide–based diaper rash ointments work quite well. If a gathered-edge diaper is the problem, the gather can be broken or a different kind of diaper used. One may need to use ½% to 1% hydrocortisone cream if the rash seems unusually inflamed, but this is not often necessary.

Ammonia burns were once fairly common causes of diaper rash. When cloth diapers and plastic or rubber diaper covers were insufficiently laundered, ammonia was sometimes produced by bacterial action on the urine. The diagnosis was straightforward: one observed a red, often slightly scaly appearance, most marked where urine contact was greatest, plus the unmistakable stench of ammonia, especially strong in the overnight diaper. Treatment required vigorous laundering and disinfection of the diapers and covers with bleach or other germicides. This old entity has largely disappeared with the availability of automatic washing machines, better detergents, and paper diapers.

Any diaper rash that fails to improve with the usual measures is likely to have an infectious component. Bacterial infections are typically small, red, pustular rashes on the buttocks and around the anus. The treatment is frequent and careful washing plus topical antibiotic cream applied a few times a day. These rashes heal very slowly. Yeast infection is much more common. It may accompany the administration of systemic antibiotics or arise for no apparent reason; in small infants, there is often a coexistent thrush. The yeast rash has a flat, red, confluent central area that often starts around the anus or the genitals, with tiny flat to raised "satellite" lesions at the periphery where the rash is extending onto healthy skin. If someone has been treating the rash with a steroid cream, the appearance will be much less red. The treatment is exposure to air and sun, frequent diaper changes, and the application of an antiyeast cream several times a day. The best are the broad-spectrum antifungal agents like clotrimazole and miconazole, which are available over the counter and labeled for use against athlete's foot. Some other antifungal agents like ciclopirox are also effective, but they are available by prescription only and are usually more expensive. Nystatin was the first reasonably effective antiyeast topical medication; it is much slower to act than the newer agents and is still available by prescription only, for no good reason. If the baby also has thrush, treat her with the same topical antifungal cream that is being used on the bottom. It should be wiped on the buccal mucosa after feedings several times a day. This is a nonstandard and much more efficacious treatment than the usual expensive, foul-tasting and wimpy nystatin liquid.

The last diaper rash entity to be aware of is the Gianotti-Crosti syndrome. This flat-topped, macular rash can start on the buttocks, but it eventually spreads to the face and extremities. The eruption is self-limited; its only importance is that it is a marker for a variety of viral infections.

🦎 TODDLER SKIN

Eczema

During the early years of childhood, eczema continues to be a major dermatologic problem. The appearance of the rash gradually evolves into a scaly, patchy dry eruption, which can be present from scalp to feet. When eczematous areas are infected, they look redder and may be weepy; old, thickened patches may also harbor a vast staphylococcal flora. Contact irritation and vigorous scratching play increasingly important roles, although food and other allergies are still crucial. In particular, house dust mite and cat allergies need to be considered. Blood tests (such as the radioallergosorbent [RAST]) for specific allergens or skin scratch tests (after about age 3 years) may clarify the causes. Cat allergy has always been difficult to manage; I have often thought that a small Mafia operation to remove offending cats would be useful. To say that families have a hard time deciding whether to keep the kid or the cat may somewhat overstate the case, but not by much. It has recently been argued that cat saliva is the specific allergen, generously spread by the kitty all over her fur and from there throughout the house. Frequent bathing of the cat plus exceedingly meticulous housekeeping, including walls, floors and furniture may be helpful. Of course, many cats run away if forced to undergo weekly baths; this may not be a bad thing. Desensitization shots are a last resort. House dust mite control has never been easy. The child's bedroom, at least, must be kept in spartan simplicity to minimize living space for the mites and to facilitate cleaning. Few families will really work hard enough at this task or persevere long enough to curtail the population of mites. The recent commercial introduction of benzoyl benzoate as a household acaricide may turn out to be useful, but my bets are on the dust mites; I think they will prevail.

Keratosis Pilaris

"What are these funny little bumps on her arms, Doctor?" If the little bumps are tiny hyperkeratotic points surrounding a minute hair, and they are on the extensor surfaces of the arms, perhaps the legs, and sometimes the cheeks, they bear the impressive name of keratosis pilaris. Most of the time, they persist for a few years in childhood, less often into adolescence and adult life. Urea cream, 10% or 20%, smooths them out temporarily, but they recur.

Insect Bites and Stings

It is remarkable how picky insects can be in their choice of victims. Families commonly relate that only a select few of their members are bitten by house spiders, fleas, or whatever. Frequently the children are favored, and insect bites in children are often dramatic in appearance. The wheal around a quite ordinary bug bite can be 3 or 4 cm in diameter, and vesiculation is by no means rare. Redness and swelling around a bee sting can extend from the foot half way to the knee and can last for days; sometimes there is even a little fever. None of this means anything; the bites are not infected. Although they itch and are tender, they rarely hurt, and no significant medical intervention is needed. First aid for insect bites is usually limited to tender loving care. Holding an ice cube to the bitten area may give everyone something harmless to do. We have had the impression that antiperspirants (which contain aluminum salts) minimize the discomfort of bee stings, but placebo-controlled studies have yet to be done. Parents may be concerned that these relatively severe local reactions may presage dangerous systemic reactions in the future; they do not. An interesting variant on insect bites is *papular urticaria,* a strange rash of papules intermixed with ordinary insect bites. It looks as if the skin were reacting in a bitelike fashion, even in areas where there were no bites. Hydroxyzine or diphenhydramine by mouth or crotamiton cream locally is comforting.

₹ MIDDLE-AGED
CHILDREN'S SKIN

Lice

Of all the small animals that infest the skin of children, the head louse, *Pediculus humanus capitis,* is the most common, the least harmful, and the most trouble. The shock, horror, and shame of the parent confronted with a lousy child must be seen and heard to be believed. The response of school teachers to an outbreak of head lice in the classroom suggests that bubonic fever cannot be far behind. A few facts should be stated: (1) Treatment of head lice can be limited to the head and the few objects directly in contact with the head, like brushes and hats. Sterilization of the entire house or surrounding city block is not indicated. Objects thought to be infested can be washed with soap and hot water, dry-cleaned, or just sealed in paper bags for 3 weeks to starve the lice to death. (2) Malathion or permethrin kills lice and nits wonderfully efficiently; one treatment nearly always suffices, but a repeat treatment 1 week later makes everyone feel better (especially the pharmacist). Lindane and pyrethrins are not as toxic to the nits; at least one and preferably two repeat treatments are a good idea. (3) It is fairly difficult to get rid of lice if the patient has dense, long, and curly hair; use malathion or permethrin for these patients. (4) If reinfestation occurs, treat the whole family. (5) A nit present on the hair shaft more than 1 cm from the scalp is either empty because the louse has already hatched or dead because it was already treated with an insecticide. A glance at the nit under the low power of your office microscope will tell you which is the case. An unhatched, live nit is worth seeing, by the way: they wiggle inside their little cocoons! The point of all this detail about nits is that school personnel sometimes demand that kids be nit free before readmission to class. This is a lot of work and a waste of time if the nits are dead. If all else fails, a vinegar rinse 15 minutes before using a nit comb will loosen them from the hair shafts.

Scabies

A worldwide epidemic of scabies has changed this from an infestation of the poor and homeless to a common problem in every social class and every age. Unlike adults, children with scabies may have infestations extending to the face. There are rarely the telltale burrows at the finger webs, often noted in adult scabies. You are most likely to be looking at a very nonspecific, finely papular, rather sparse, and highly pruritic rash, which you have already treated with a steroid that didn't help. Treatment needs to be carried out precisely, as follows. (1) Every contact should be treated. (2) Sheets, pillow cases, and clothes should be hot-laundered. Anything not washable should be dry-cleaned. (3) Permethrin 5% (not the 1% lotion used for lice) should be applied at bedtime. The skin should be clean, cool, and dry; it should not be applied immediately after a hot bath. The medication should cover the body from soles to scalp. It should be washed off the next morning. (4) Warn the family that neither the rash nor the itching will improve for days; the scabies mites will be dead, but their bodies and their metabolic products will remain in the skin. No new lesions will appear. Repeated application of permethrin is not needed, but oral antipruritics may be used. (5) Recurrences of scabies usually mean continued exposure to an untreated case.

Impetigo

Children's skin generally does a good job of resisting bacterial infection. When you see impetigo, there are often extra factors that have allowed the germs to break through the ordinary barriers. A chronic bacterial nasal discharge will suffice. Hot, muggy weather also increases the incidence and virulence of impetigo. The combination of casual hygiene and multiple abrasions characteristic of small boys in summertime explains a good many cases. Family or classroom outbreaks are the exception; impetigo is not particularly contagious. The precise roles played by beta streptococcus and *Staphylococcus* have exercised investigators for years. It is clear that bullous impetigo is a staphylococcal infection. It needs to be treated aggressively with antistaphylococcal antibiotics like first-generation cephalosporins, amoxicillin-clavulanate, or dicloxacillin. Other forms of impetigo may be streptococcal, staphylococcal, or both. Before the advent of mupirocin topical cream, it was useful to culture the lesions. Streptococcal impetigo had to be treated with a systemic antibiotic, usually penicillin; *Staphylococcus* would respond slowly but surely to local bacitracin or bacitracin-polymyxin ointment. However, mupirocin does a nice job of fighting against either pathogen or both pathogens; unless the disease is widespread or unusually virulent, it is enough to proceed with mupirocin and skip the expense of the skin cultures. I really hate to say this, however; it offends my need to know what I'm treating.

Hot-Tub Folliculitis

Now here is a disease of affluence! This papular, truncal eruption is a *Pseudomonas* infection spread in hot water. Topical polymyxin or triple antibiotic ointment is curative—and keep that kid out of the hot tub.

Molluscum Contagiosum

The viral infection known as molluscum contagiosum is also spread in water. The lesions start as tiny, less than 1 mm in diameter, papules and mature into 1- to 2-mm firm, pearly to pink papules, most of which have a clearly umbilicated center. You may need a magnifying lens for the examination; the otoscope works fairly well, but a pocket 10× lens is preferable. The natural history of molluscum is interesting. The rash may remain confined to a few lesions, or it may spread widely with hundreds of papules. Redness may develop around a few of the papules; this is a skin reaction that may precede the spontaneous disappearance of the entire eruption. Sometimes the lesions disappear rapidly without preceding inflammatory response. There are three management options: (1) watchful waiting; (2) manual removal of each lesion by popping it out of the skin with a #20 hollow needle (it hardly hurts at all, honest!); and (3) touching each lesion with a drop of cantharidin 0.7% solution, which causes a small blister to form under and around the molluscum. This may need to be repeated a few times as new lesions become large enough to see.

Warts

The wart virus seems to require a degree of cooperation from the human host. The common sites of infection on hands and feet suggest that only abraded or otherwise traumatized skin is likely to be infected. The rarity of warts on adult skin suggests that some kind of immunity to wart infection eventually develops with age. If common warts are left alone, the majority will disappear, although it may take some years for this to happen. If neither the child nor his parents are unduly alarmed by the wart, and if it is not in a place where it causes discomfort, the best treatment is no treatment at all. A wart that catches on clothing and bleeds, a wart on the plantar surface of the foot that hurts because it is walked on, or a wart that is distorting a fingernail or toenail—all these are candidates for removal.

The reason to avoid therapy, if possible, is that none of the available options is very satisfactory. Freezing the wart with liquid nitrogen is certainly the fastest cure; unfortunately; it hurts a good bit, especially if the wart is large and even more if it is a deep, plantar growth. Cantharidin solution carefully applied to the wart forms a blister within or under the wart; 2 weeks after the first treatment, the dead material is débrided and more cantharidin is applied. As many as four treatments may be needed. This method often causes a large, painful, and even hemorrhagic reaction; furthermore, one may end up with a ring of new warts around the old lesion. Home application of salicylic or lactic acid eventually cures most warts; the nightly ritual of soaking, débridement, and medication is daunting; many patients give up long before the wart does.

A painless and charming wart treatment is self-cure by visualization, a sort of self-hypnosis. It has been known at least since the 1920s that hypnosis can change the rate of healing of skin wounds, and for centuries there has been a plethora of traditional folk remedies for warts, which seem to rely on suggestion. It should therefore not be too surprising that warts be cured quite nicely by the patient herself. The technique is simple. (1) Get a timing device like a 2-minute egg timer. (2) Go to a quiet and private place where your little brother will not interrupt and make fun of you. (3) Look at the wart and imagine that it is becoming smaller and disappearing. Keep this up for 2 minutes; when your attention wanders from the wart, and it will, just resume visualizing. (4) Repeat twice daily, if possible.

Families report several outcomes for self-cure by visualization. The child who thought this was a dumb idea at the outset abandons the treatment within a few days. A few children give up after 1 or 2 weeks. The large majority of children who were intrigued or excited at the beginning persevere; their warts generally disappear quite abruptly after 6 to 8 weeks. The sense of delighted self-mastery that these kids earn is wonderful. The disadvantage for the practitioner is that word will get around in your medical community that you cure warts by witchcraft; in some settings this may be embarrassing. (I should add that this treatment was devised and taught to me by a 9-year-old patient. He had accompanied a friend to a hypnotist who was treating his friend's warts. Peter decided that he could accomplish the same thing for himself without anyone's help, and he did.)

Tinea Corporis

Laboratory help in the diagnosis of tinea corporis should be easy and inexpensive, but that is not always the case. Potassium hydroxide preparations of skin scrapings can be difficult to interpret; dermatophyte test medium (DTM) cultures don't always grow. So from time to time you will make a clinical diagnosis based on the appearance of slightly red, more or less round skin patches with a scaly periphery and a hint of clearing in the center. Several such lesions of various sizes, plus a history of dog or cat contact will make your impression even more comfortably founded. The imidazole topical antifungal agents work slowly but effectively; only if there are vast numbers or continuing crops of lesions need you consider oral griseofulvin. If you use griseofulvin, choose the ultramicrosized preparation; it is much better absorbed.

Tinea Pedis

For some reason, the conventional teaching about tinea pedis has been that babies and small children don't get it. Unfortunately, the conventional teaching is wrong: they do get it. This is yet another example of the wisdom of one of my medical school teachers who told us that at least half of what we were being taught was incorrect; unfortunately, nobody knew which half. Fungal infections seem to thrive on feet that are kept warm and sweaty; the inside of a modern shoe made largely of rubber and plastics is fungus heaven. Add to that socks made of nonabsorbent synthetic thread, and it is a surprise that our feet don't rot off to our ankles. Some kids clearly have very sweaty feet, even in better-ventilated settings, and some families have a long tradition of chronic tinea pedis. These are the children most likely to have athlete's foot infections in infancy.

It is important to differentiate tinea pedis from eczema and contact dermatitis of the foot. An eczema usually involves the ankles or the dorsal portion of the midfoot. A contact dermatitis looks like a superficial burn and covers the portions of the toes and feet most exposed to shoe chemicals. The toe webs are spared. Tinea pedis usually is most obvious as scaling and maceration of the toe webs, especially the most lateral webs. There may also be the pattern of red, finely vesicular, itchy lesions along the edges of the sole. Chronic tinea pedis may cause diffuse scaling of the entire sole, especially in older children. Because host factors of diminished resistance and increased sweatiness are important and because most children's footwear does not ventilate the foot, tinea pedis tends to recur. Going barefoot, wearing sandals, choosing socks made of light wool or cotton, using absorbent foot powders—all these techniques may help control the disease. Treatment with any imidazole antifungal cream twice a day leads to rapid improvement; several weeks may be needed for complete clearing.

Tinea Unguium

Toenail fungus infections are truly rare in early childhood. This is fortunate because treatment is wholly unsatisfactory. If the nail is trimmed short and filed or ground down as thin as possible, a modest degree of control may be achieved by naftifine gel or ciclopirox cream every day. As soon as you stop treatment, the nail infection usually reappears. The same is true of systemic treatment with griseofulvin; the nails look great after 6 to 12 months of medication, but relapse after treatment is nearly universal. Oral ketoconazole may work better than griseofulvin, but it not infrequently causes liver injury and occasionally kills people, which seems like a heavy price to pay for pretty toenails. Sometimes the wisest course is to do nothing, offensive as that may be to our sense of medical omnipotence.

Tinea Versicolor

This superficial fungus infection is caused by a quite different organism, *Malassezia furfur (Pityrosporon orbiculare)*, which seems to need skin oil to thrive. I've seen it only in pre-teens and adolescents, but it is said to occur in young infants as well. The lesions are not very dramatic: rather faint macules gradually increasing in size to blotches several centimeters in diameter, slightly pink or tan at first and then often pale and depigmented, and sometimes a bit itchy. Since tinea versicolor tends to start on the back, it is easily overlooked and ignored even by its host. Initial treatment is easy: daily shampooing with selenium sulfide 2.5% or zinc pyrithione 1% to 2% for a week or two. The imidazole antifungal creams also work well, but their cost becomes prohibitive because large areas are usually involved. The itching and pinkness disappear promptly, but the depigmentation may persist until sun exposure occurs. The major problem with tinea versicolor is recurrence. The organism is ubiquitous, and some people's skin gets infected again and again. A degree of control can be obtained by a routine of weekly shampooing with either of these agents, at least during the warm seasons of the year, when recurrences are most common.

Psoriasis

I am always surprised by psoriasis, and I miss the diagnosis more times than not. In children, psoriasis often starts unimpressively, just a patch or two of moderately scaly, slightly reddened skin. One thinks of eczema, a small contact irritation, or perhaps tinea corporis. The nice, characteristic, silvery-scaled, rather raised plaques may not appear for many months. Another presentation may be a widespread, papular eruption that does not look at all like "classic" psoriasis. In any event, I end up asking for help from a dermatologist. Treatment is often complex and always prolonged; if it involves tars, anthralin, etretinate, and ultraviolet treatments, the dermatologists should handle it.

Contact Dermatitis, Including Poison Ivy and Oak

Kids' skin is quite tough, and not a great many substances are likely to cause contact irritations. *Toxicodendron,* formerly *Rhus,* dermatitis (poison ivy and poison oak) probably causes the most trouble. One also sees metal allergy from the nickel alloyed to silver and gold jewelry; cosmetic reactions, especially from eye makeup; a variety of chemical irritations from footwear; and a kind of chronic eczematoid irritation from dishwashing detergent. For most ordinary and mild cases, avoidance of the irritant plus treatment with 1% hydrocortisone cream allows prompt healing.

Poison oak and poison ivy are different from other types of contact dermatitis. There is an important element of sensitization as well as plain contact irritation. The reaction may be exceedingly widespread, prolonged, and severe. The folklore surrounding this disease is impressive and uniformly misleading. Families need to know that the offending oleoresin becomes fixed to the skin within minutes to hours. Delayed bathing will not remove it. Watching the eruptions appear at more and more sites over a few days leads to the mistaken notion that the patient is spreading it by scratching, but this is not the case. Factors such as differing skin thicknesses, the dose of oleoresin, and probably local skin sensitivity affect the rate of development of lesions. It usually takes 2 to 3 days to break out after poison oak or ivy exposure, but the individual who has had previous episodes may develop a severe reaction within less than 24 hours.

In a minimal case the lesions are red macules, papules, and scratches that are few in number and not weepy or blistered. A mild steroid such as 1% hydrocortisone can be used several times a day.

More severe cases can sometimes be managed with class 1 or 2 steroid ointments, used sparingly, plus an oral antipruritic (hydroxyzine or diphenhydramine). However, severe cases tend to be quite widespread, and the amount of steroid cream needed becomes exceedingly costly. With the strongest local steroids, absorption and consequent suppression of the pituitary-adrenal axis are another consideration. In these instances, it makes more sense to use oral prednisone for about 1 week, rarely for a little longer. I start with 1 to 2 mg/kg/day divided into three doses, and I taper the dose as soon as the rash is improving, usually by about the third day. Even with the use of prednisone, the patient will gain some benefit from local steroids and oral antipruritics during the first few days. I ask the family to call if there is not prompt diminishing of the rash and discomfort; a follow-up visit is rarely needed. It is worthwhile to teach these kids how to recognize and therefore have a chance to avoid their local variety of *Toxicodendron*. Hyposensitization treatments with orally administered extracts have not been impressively successful but should be considered for the patient with severe sensitivity and frequent recurrences.

❧ ADOLESCENT SKIN

Acne

The treatment of adolescent acne starts when the adolescent wants it to. You may notice the first crops of comedones, and the parents may ask you to prescribe for the 12-year-old's pustules, but nothing happens until the patient himself decides to take action. From then on, what happens bears only a glancing similarity to good medical practice. Acne therapy is, regrettably, in the hands of the peer culture and the advertisers of cosmetics.

When the teenager does decide that the doctor should be involved in this process, provide the information needed for understanding. I use a hand-out (Appendix B), one copy each to patient and parent, and review it with the patient, highlighting the pertinent parts.

My general guidelines are as follows:

1. Keep it simple, at least at first. Twice-a-day routines are nearly always ignored or forgotten at the beginning, when the "magical cure" is still anticipated.

2. Find out what the current acne-control routine has been; it may guide your choices.

3. Start gently; if your prescription causes unpleasant side effects, you will lose credibility.

4. To clear comedones, use tretinoin (Retin-A); start with the cream (0.05%) for the fairest-skinned patients or the gel (0.01%), to be used every 2 to 3 nights; increase slowly to every night. Re-check in about 2 months, and increase the strength if necessary.

5. To control pustules and decrease skin oiliness, use benzoyl peroxide 5% aqueous gel; if drying is not needed, use a topical antibiotic (tetracycline, clindamycin, or erythromycin).

6. When infection is a major problem, use an oral antibiotic instead: (a) *tetracycline* (cheap; if the patient cannot remember to take it 1 or 2 hours away from mealtime—and none of them can—just increase the dose), started at 500 mg b.i.d. and decreased to once daily after a few months; (b) *doxycycline* (expensive, but absorption is not interfered with by milk or food), 50 mg b.i.d. or 100 mg daily, later decreased to 50 mg daily; (c) *erythromycin estolate* (expensive and often causes nausea if given before a meal), 250 b.i.d. or t.i.d., later decreased to 250 mg daily. Oral antibiotics are wonderfully useful; it may be necessary to use rather generous doses for years, and the remarkably low incidence of side effects, especially of the tetracyclines, makes this possible. Resistance of involved skin bacteria is an uncommon problem.

7. Tretinoin HS, benzoyl peroxide AM, and an oral antibiotic once or twice a day will eventually be needed for many cases.

8. Scrubs, pads, alcohol-based drying agents, sulfur, resorcinol, and other topical agents have very little place in acne treatment.

9. Isotretinoin is exceedingly effective for severe, cystic acne. Because of its toxicity, I think it should be left to dermatologists, if at all possible. Techniques such as intralesional injections and freezing are also within their province, rather than ours.

10. The biggest unsolved problem of acne therapy is follow-up; you really need to see them after about 2 months to tailor your treatment to the initial response. When the acne eventually worsens as adolescence progresses, you will want to see them again. Unfortunately, the teenagers often change to advertised over-the-counter nostrums or drift off to the dermatologists, who then have the same problems of noncompliance.

❧ CHAPTER 18

Minor Injuries

How you decide to manage children's minor injuries depends on a number of factors. Are you next door to an emergency room? Do you have adequate equipment for handling lacerations, sprains, and burns? Do you have office space that can be tied up for the hour or so it may take to clean, débride, and suture a wound? Is your office safe enough at night for you to meet a family and treat an injury? At the Berkeley Pediatric Group, we decided years ago to manage injuries, whenever possible, at our office. We have the space, we have the equipment, and it is a safe neighborhood. Furthermore, we wanted to avoid the use of emergency rooms. They are frightening places for kids, full of strange sights and horrifying sounds. These days they have become wildly overcrowded and unbelievably expensive. So we tell families to call us when there is an injury, day or night. Screening over the telephone is easy. We decide whether the services of the hospital and its staff are likely to be needed, and 9 times out of 10 we have the child brought to our office instead. The disadvantage for the physician is that one may end up repairing a laceration late at night in the office and wishing one had an emergency room nurse handy to help. Nevertheless, it is comforting for the child and parents to be cared for in a familiar place by a familiar doctor.

The investment in supplies and equipment is not inconsiderable. You need to be able to clean and close wounds, dress burns, and treat sprains. For the unexpected major emergency you need oxygen and masks; intravenous fluids, needles, and lines; a laryngoscope and endotracheal tubes; and a variety of emergency drugs for the treatment of anaphylaxis, asthma, convulsions, and severe pain. It is also neces-

187

sary to train office staff in emergency management; cardiopulmonary resuscitation training is a must. An occasional practice run in handling the more important emergencies is a good idea.

Abrasions and Lacerations

The most common injuries you will see are soft tissue abrasions and lacerations. Appropriate cleansing is often the most uncomfortable part for the child. It is less painful to rinse and wash with saline instead of water. If an injury is fairly extensive and especially if it looks like suturing will be needed, I sometimes anesthetize the area first and clean it up later. Topical use of 4% lidocaine solution on the surface of an abrasion may suffice. The recent introduction of tetracaine, adrenaline, and cocaine (TAC) topical anesthesia to replace injection anesthesia is attractive, but because the solution is unstable, requires frequent replacement, and is exceedingly expensive, we have not adopted it. The use of adhesive strips instead of sutures is a great help if certain guidelines are followed. The skin must be completely clean; even a little skin oil defeats the adhesive. Use soap and water, followed by alcohol or acetone on the intact skin near the laceration. Never try to use adhesive strips on the chin; the combination of constant motion and intermittent saliva, food, and drink rapidly loosens the strips. Do not use them on any area where constant flexing will occur, such as the knee. If the area cannot be immobilized, the strips will fail. Lacerations parallel to the flexion lines of the skin are the easiest to close with strips. Lacerations across skin lines tend to pull apart. Adhesive strips are most successful on the scalp, on the forehead (for horizontal cuts only), around the eyes, on the forearms, and on the hands and feet. Small lacerations of the digits are particularly well-suited to adhesive strip repair, especially if adequate immobilization is obtained.

Sprains

FINGERS

Ball injuries are the most common cause of sprained fingers. The major pitfall in their treatment is the possibility of an associated avulsed tendon. Examination should be aimed at assessing muscle and tendon competence. X-ray examination to exclude a fracture is rarely needed. The usual finger sprain is treated quite simply with immobilization by strapping the injured finger in a gently flexed curve to the neighboring digit. Several pieces of ½-inch-wide heavy cloth adhesive tape are used. The injured joint should be held firmly enough to discourage movement. Teach the family how to replace the tapes as they become loose or disgustingly filthy. About 3 to 5 days of taping usually suffices. Sometimes the sprain is painful enough to warrant ibuprofen for a day or so.

ANKLES

Most sprained ankles are straightforward and easily dealt with, but a severe sprain may hide a small fracture or even an avulsed tendon. For this reason, I like to recheck ankle sprains in a few days to assure myself that all is going well. I lean on the teenagers to give their sprains enough time to heal before returning to full and unsupported activity, because recurrent sprains can become a major dilemma. Initial treatment requires rest, elevation, and immobilization. It seems to me that ice helps control pain and swelling if used promptly after an acute sprain, but I am unconvinced that fancy regimens of alternating ice and heat accomplish anything afterward. This is an area of folklore elevated to orthopedic mythology. Crutches plus heavy elastic bandaging plus gradual resumption of weight-bearing used to be routine for severe ankle sprains. Now, air-filled or gel-filled "casts" have made early ambulation and weight-bearing possible. Crutches are now needed only rarely and briefly. Whenever crutches are used, the patient should be shown how to hold the crutches firmly, with the forearms extended and the top of the crutches resting against the lateral chest wall, rather than tucked up into the axilla. Weight should be borne by the upper extremities, not the axilla.

Dislocated Radial Head ("Nursemaid's Elbow")

Should this be renamed "Au pair's dislocation?" The main point with a dislocated radial head is to minimize both diagnosis and treatment. All too often these children are subjected to radiographic studies when simple clinical examination should suffice. The story of the injury may not always be available, but the picture of the sad-faced little child standing in your office with her arm dangling limply at her side or held carefully by the other hand is close to pathognomonic. Oddly enough, both child and parent may think that the injury is at the wrist, but careful palpation nearly always clarifies the picture. The crucial maneuver in replacing the radial head is supination of the forearm. This can be done easily by grasping the child's hand in a handshake position, stabilizing the elbow with one's other hand and simultaneously supinating the hand while flexing the elbow. At the conclusion of the movement the child's palm nearly touches her shoulder. It may require two or three such motions before the radial head slips back into the annular ligament and one feels and hears a click. Some clinicians use a combined supination and extension of the forearm instead; this is apparently equally effective. After what seems to be a successful reduction, the child is kept in the office for 10 or 15 minutes. By that time, nearly every child is playing happily, using both arms comfortably. Any immobilization or other intervention is wholly unnecessary. If reduction cannot be accomplished or if the child continues to complain of discomfort and refuses to use her arm, it is time for an x-ray film and possibly an orthopedist.

Whenever I see a child with a dislocated radial head, I explain the problem to the parent and note that recurrences are common. If a second dislocation occurs, I can usually instruct the parent over the telephone to reduce the dislocation. A few parents find this too frightening to attempt, but the majority succeed and are delighted with their accomplishment.

Minor Burns

Most of the burns sustained by children are first-degree or superficial second-degree in depth. When large areas of skin are involved, pain and fluid loss are important to manage, and these injuries often require hospital care. Deep second-degree burns may be difficult to distinguish from full-thickness third-degree burns; consultation with a burn specialist may be useful.

For most minor burns, gentle cleansing with saline, plus soap if necessary, is followed by application of an occlusive dressing. The dressing can be any of several ointments (bacitracin, bacitracin-polymyxin, petrolatum, povidone-iodine, or silver sulfadiazine) covered with gauze and held in place with paper tape. If the burn is small and the burn site is unlikely to be traumatized, open care without the gauze cover is a possibility. However, most burns hurt much less once they are protected by a substantial dressing. Unless an extremely heavy layer of ointment is used, the dressing will unfailingly adhere to the wound. Change the dressing the next day before this happens, and redress as often as needed to keep the wound surface from further injury by the bandage. A variety of materials have been devised to allow healing without adherence. A simple plastic membrane (Telfa) works moderately well. The newer artificial membrane dressings (e.g., Omniderm, Duoderm) seem to be superior in allowing rapid healing, but they are exceedingly expensive; since these minor burns heal so nicely anyway, it is hard to justify their use.

Subungual Hematomas

Fingernail and toenail injuries sufficient to cause subungual bleeding cry out for treatment. If blood remains under the nail, it continues to be painful for many days. Relief is obtained by placing a hole in the nail either with a special battery driven drill or by melting a hole with repeated gentle touches with a red-hot paper clip. Either a Bunsen burner or a small alcohol lamp may be used to heat the bent paper clip, which one holds with a clamp. At the instant the nail is penetrated, a geyser of blood erupts and the pain is gone. If you are sufficiently careful, neither instrument will touch the nail bed. Using the little drill looks much more scientific and perhaps less frightening, but the old paper clip method works just fine.

Epistaxes

An acute nosebleed may have an obvious cause, usually trauma, or may be apparently spontaneous, in which case a cause must be sought. Low-grade nasal infection, dry air, high altitudes, and nose-rubbing or nose-picking (which can have an allergic basis) are the usual factors. Recurrent epistaxes raise the possibility of an underlying bleeding disorder. Treatment of most nosebleeds is exceedingly simple but rarely done correctly. In the vast majority of cases, the source of blood is the venous plexus overlying the cartilage of the nasal septum. Direct pressure should be used to collapse these venous channels by squeezing between thumb and forefinger the entire anterior, cartilaginous part of the nose. Bleeding will stop instantly if enough of the nose is compressed. Use your fingers; Kleenex, handkerchiefs and gauze pads just get in the way. Keep the pressure up without stopping for 5 to 10 minutes; it takes time for clotting to occur. If the patient is supine, venous pressure in the head will be a bit higher and bleeding more copious, so keep the patient upright if possible. Ice applied anywhere on the head is supposed to cause vasoconstriction in the nose; if someone can hold ice on the nape of the patient's neck, this may be moderately helpful.

A severe and persistent bleed may require the use of topical phenylephrine 0.5% or 1% solution or silver nitrate cauterization. Silver nitrate hurts; use a local anesthetic like 4% lidocaine topical solution first. Packing with an absorbable material like Oxycel or the old-fashioned but effective piece of bacon fat may rarely be necessary. Recurrent bleeds can often be prevented by using a hydrocortisone-antibiotic ointment twice a day for a few weeks.

Poisonings

The first words to say about poisonings are prevention, prevention, and prevention. This means that practitioners dealing with children have to invest time and energy in teaching families about the risks of toxic ingestion and the various strategies for minimizing them. I tell parents which household and garden materials are poisonous, stressing especially cleansers, disinfectants, polishes, hydrocarbons, lye, drugs, and garden chemicals and plants. Then I urge them to throw away every poison that they do not really need. Household disinfectants are truly useless, liquid furniture polishes can be replaced with foams and pastes, and drugs no longer needed should be discarded. Some garden chemicals are needlessly dangerous, and less hazardous substitutes can be used instead. Safe storage of dangerous substances is easy to advise but may be hard to accomplish. For real protection, a locked cabinet out of the reach of young children is ideal; it is also usually impossible for families to arrange. Especially in dysfunctional and chaotic households, it is unlikely that a truly safe environment can be maintained. Even in the best-regulated homes, disruptions of routine occur because of illness, visitors, moving, and the like. During these times, poisonings are increasingly common.

Syrup of ipecac is the second line of defense. My guess is that it takes an average of two or three requests from me before the little bottle is purchased. Ipecac will do no good unless all the adult caretakers know about its existence and whereabouts. We do not recommend having activated charcoal at home; it is sometimes the best treatment but it is exceedingly difficult to administer. In our area, telephone calls by families to hospital emergency rooms and poison control centers too often result in overtreatment. We prefer to be called instead; if our office library fails to guide us in managing an ingestion, we call the poison center ourselves. The vast majority of childhood ingestions involve substances (usually cosmetics, soaps, detergents, and plants) with little or no toxicity. Furthermore, many of the toxic substances are taken in insignificant amounts, warranting no treatment. The few remaining significant ingestions are usually handled initially by telephone; follow-up can be done in the office or by telephone, depending on the circumstances. We use a separate, colored sheet of paper for our chart record of ingestions, and we note all the facts in full detail. More than one of these poison papers in a child's record is a literal red flag.

Pain Relief

The pain of acute injury is easy to relieve, but we have to remember to treat it. Sometimes we focus so much on the definitive therapy of the injury itself that we overlook the child's continuing discomfort. Nondrug methods of pain control include immobilization, ice, occlusive dressings, and tender loving care; each has a role. Drug use obviously depends on the nature and severity of the pain. Aspirin is still a useful minor analgesic. In the absence of chicken pox or influenza, you need not worry about Reye syndrome. The palatability of aspirin in the children's chewable form is a great help, especially with kids who reject acetaminophen. The anti-inflammatory effect is probably an additional help in children with burns and soft tissue injuries. Acetaminophen has equal efficacy in pain control without anti-inflammatory effect. Ibuprofen is a somewhat more powerful analgesic, and it has a significant anti-inflammatory effect if used in full doses. The liquid forms require a prescription and are expensive; over-the-counter generic tablets are relatively cheap. Like other nonsteroidal anti-inflammatory drugs, ibuprofen has more toxicity than aspirin or acetaminophen, but this is rarely a problem for short-term use in children.

Codeine is a great drug for pain. Especially when used along with aspirin or acetaminophen, codeine controls the discomfort of most severe soft tissue injuries and even some fracture pain. The easiest way to prescribe codeine for small children is in the form of liquid cough syrups like promethazine with codeine. These don't taste too terrible, require no triplicate form, and are often already available in the home medicine cabinet. For older children, use aspirin and codeine or acetaminophen with codeine tablets. A dose to control pain will be about twice as much as you would use for cough control; use about 2 to 4 mg/kg/day, divided every 3 to 4 hours for small children, 15 to 60 mg every 3 to 4 hours for older kids.

For severe pain from fractures and burns, morphine or meperidine (Demerol) is required. Be generous; there is literally no risk of addiction when you treat acute pain in childhood. If repeated doses are needed, give them before the pain gets bad; there is no discernible virtue in needless suffering.

CHAPTER 19

The Management of Everyday Illnesses

A few years ago the dean of a western medical school spent his sabbatical year practicing medicine away from the ivory tower. At the conclusion of this refreshing and unusual experience he reported to his faculty that a great deal of his time was spent in the management of illness. He seemed to have been surprised. By "management" he meant the ongoing totality of illness care, including the processes of diagnosis, the undertaking of treatment, and the subsequent follow-up of the patient's course. He was certainly correct; it is what we do, and it does feel like more than the sum of its parts. In this chapter, we take a look at some of the more interesting and neglected aspects of management: using the office laboratory, when to treat and when to watch, where to treat—hospital or home, and the tactics of drug use.

The Laboratory and the Diagnostic Process

It is instructive to watch the changes in one's medical practices over time and equally interesting to observe how one's partners approach identical problems. I've noticed that I tend to use the lab less and less. When I was first in practice, the ambiguity of clinical situations left me exceedingly anxious, and my response was often to look for a clarifying test. The number of STAT white blood cell counts my patients underwent was astounding. I never reached the point of carrying a microscope in the car to have it available on house calls, as one friend of mine did, but I certainly depended on the lab. My partners leaned in different directions: one of them used sedimentation rates

195

the way I used the white blood cell count. As I watched his management of cases, it became clear that his sedimentation rate determina-
tions rarely, if ever, changed his understanding of the problem or his
subsequent treatment of the child. As I watched my own cases it
became equally clear that I was learning precious little from my white
cell counts. The same turned out to be true for nasopharyngeal cultures, routine complete blood counts in children past infancy, and
x-ray films of sprained ankles and bumped heads. I don't mean to
imply that lab studies are useless; far from it. They can be a great
help in clarifying the clinical problem, but one's expectations should
be modest. In our office lab, we do only the tests required often
enough to keep the lab technicians practiced in their performance; we
limit ourselves further to tests that are helpful to have immediately
on hand for the convenience of our patients and ourselves. Getting
the result of a urinalysis in 5 minutes and the urine culture overnight
beats sending our patient across town to the hospital lab and waiting
indefinitely for the answers.

Here is our current office lab repertoire (subject to whatever
changes will be imposed by the developing federal rules):

Hematology. The automatic counter provides a complete blood
count and indices; the differential and platelet counts are done
by hand. It would be nice to be able to afford a machine to do
these, too, but one would still often want a smear for mor-
phology.

Urinalysis. The complicated and expensive dipsticks are wonderful; they replace microscopic examinations if the dipstick is negative. The indicators of leukocyte esterase and nitrite are a great
help in screening for infection. See the chapter on urinary tract
infection for details on urine collection and culturing.

Bacteriology. We culture throats, noses (but not often), urine
(using a calibrated loop rather than a pipette), skin (for bacteria,
fungi, yeasts), and vulva and vagina for bacteria other than *Neisseria gonorrhoeae* and *Chlamydia* (we send those out). The rapid
Streptococcus tests are not wholly satisfactory but we do a few
of them. We do potassium hydroxide preparations for fungi,
wet preparations for *Trichomonas,* and sticky tape preparations

for pinworms. We can do blood cultures, but we generally send these to a hospital lab. Stool for ova and parasites are too rarely done: we send them out.

Miscellaneous. We do the mononucleosis spot test, Streptozyme (rarely useful), theophylline blood levels, pregnancy tests, occult blood in stool, nasal smears for eosinophils and polys.

When I think about what tests to do, I try to balance the urgency of the clinical situation with the costs to the family, which include the discomfort and anxiety of the child, the inconvenience for the parents, and the money that someone will have to pay. Most of the time you can proceed deliberately and sequentially. If you think the sore throat is possibly a streptococcal infection and the patient is not particularly ill, a throat culture is all that is needed. More often than not, the culture is negative and the child is much improved when you call the family the next day. If the culture is negative and the illness persists, you can re-examine the child and consider getting a complete blood count and a mononucleosis test. On the other hand, you would proceed much more aggressively if the child were quite ill or if the teenager had final exams starting the next day.

This leads to a general consideration of how one thinks diagnostically. The current fad of algorithms seems to be based on the notion that the diagnostic process mimics the workings of a computer program, that is, lots of choice points where one can proceed logically in either of two directions. I think we work in a much freer and fuzzier fashion. As I hear the history of an illness or a complaint unfolding from patient or parent (or both), I'm looking for patterns. Some patterns are simple: the acute strep throat that hits hard and fast, accompanied by a bellyache and a headache, is a good example. Some are idiosyncratic: the child whose sore throats are nearly always streptococcal, no matter how mild the complaints and bland-appearing the physical exam. Another child always has a sore throat with every illness, but never, ever has a strep throat. I'm also factoring in the tendency of some children to run high fevers with every trivial bug, the anxiety about illness that distorts some parents' perceptions, and the denial that clouds the reports of others.

As I proceed with the exam, hypotheses are forming and being discarded, and by the end of the process there is usually a likely diagnosis at hand or one to be confirmed. Less often, there is a differential diagnosis list. Once in a while there is pure confusion. This may mean that the disease process has not yet revealed itself. Remember the old medical aphorism: "Fortunate is the physician who sees the patient last." It may mean that I have missed something important in the history or the exam; it may mean that this is a real zebra and I can't see the stripes; most often it means that emotional factors are present and not clearly expressed. This can be summarized as **Grossman's Law of Difficult Diagnosis: The patient with multisystem symptoms and no findings is a lot more likely to be suffering from depression than from dermatomyositis.**

Treating and Waiting

What happens at this point is what medical management is all about. I mentioned the role of parental anxiety in muddying the waters of diagnosis. The physician's anxiety is at least as important, as decisions are made about the appropriate steps to be taken. Our anxiety will be influenced by how clearly we see the entire process. As clinical experience is gained and pattern recognition improves, we learn when we can relax and do nothing. The favorite diagnosis of one of my senior partners was "Little bug," which meant that the affliction before her was un-nameable but basically unimportant. When I first joined our group and noted this common entry on her charts, I was somewhat taken aback by the casual imprecision; eventually I saw it as calm wisdom. The Britishism "masterful inactivity" conveys the same approach: one can sometimes simply watch and wait. Does this seem dangerous and untenable in the present medical environment of litigious patients? Perhaps so; a patient recently told me that her former obstetrician in another part of the country had answered a medical question by saying, "I'll be able to tell you after I've checked with my lawyer." However, here in Berkeley we still have the option of watchful waiting when you trust yourself and the family trusts you.

The contrast with the hospital setting is interesting. In the teaching hospital, a differential diagnosis should be and is produced, and lab studies are often undertaken to explore several diagnostic possibilities simultaneously. This may result from the necessity to move quickly because of the severity of the clinical problem or to minimize the length of the hospital stay; it may also reflect the defensive necessity of protection from criticism. Perhaps the hardest course to follow is simple observation.

The other contrast between inpatient and outpatient management is the loneliness of outpatient care. The house officer in the teaching center is surrounded by colleagues and superiors, supported by the knowledge that other eyes watch his patients and other minds consider their problems. He relies on experienced nurses to correct at least some of his errors and bring him new information about changes in his patient's condition. He can quickly (sometimes too quickly) obtain consultation from specialists. Even in the small hours of the night, he knows he is not completely alone. This is not so for the community practitioner caring for a patient at home. The telephone rings at 3:00 A.M.; I listen to the description of the symptoms, consider the likely possibilities and the worst ones, decide that the child can be treated with an antipyretic (or a cough suppressant or clear fluids), give my advice, and turn out the light. I lie in bed wondering what I have missed. *Haemophilus influenzae* septicemia? Is it spasmodic croup or the start of epiglottitis? An early meningitis? A retrocecal appendicitis? I suspect all of us have our own lists of favorite worries. Practice in a small group like ours helps a lot. "Come have a look at this rash." "Hey, have you noticed we're seeing some nasty viral croups?" "Do you think we should be giving up amoxicillin for sinusitis?" "I'm worried about this kid with fever and a high white count." However, much of the time you are on you own, carrying the full burden of decisions and finding it a considerable load.

One solution is to get consultations often and early; I find this very difficult to do. Perhaps it is because we pediatricians were trained to do everything by ourselves back in the 1950s. The prideful habit of pretended omniscience has died slowly in me. I still find it hard to admit to myself or to a family that I need the opinion of an ear, nose, and throat specialist or a dermatology or allergy consultant. A tempting but unwise solution is to use the hospital as an unadmitted source of consultative assistance, counting on the house staff and the ward attending to back one up. The problem with this is the inevitable confusion about who is in charge; better to bite the bullet and ask for help when you want it.

Treatment at Home or in Hospital

Needless to say, there are plenty of good reasons for putting a patient in the hospital. Without enumerating these reasons, I suggest that one consider the hospital as a tool of considerable power, the use of which carries risks and awesome expense, to be used when a specific task is to be accomplished. If the task can be done without the hospital, that alternative may be worth considering. The outpatient management of serious illness is difficult and time-consuming; don't embark on it lightly. It requires a trained office staff, colleagues committed to the process, cooperative and able parents, and available lab services. The advantages are vastly reduced expense, avoidance of separation of children from their parents during a stressful time, decreased risk of hospital-acquired disease, and usually less emotional upset for all concerned. Our group has done home phototherapy for hyperbilirubinemia since 1974; we have done home treatment of septic joints, osteomyelitis, severe asthma, freshly diagnosed diabetes, and peritonsillar abscesses. One pediatrician from a nearby community teases me every time we meet at Children's Hospital: "Why, I thought you folks at Berkeley Pediatric Group *never* admitted a patient here." Maybe we take this a bit far. One of our newer partners told me how frightened she had been when treating a teenager with a peritonsillar abscess as an outpatient. "But I thought we *had* to, in the group." Carrying the responsibility of home treatment can also be too stressful for the family; one needs to assess this in every case, and sometimes home therapy must be abandoned.

The Use of Drugs

Treatment of childhood illness means medicines, more often than not. Even though many illnesses pass without any medical intervention, we often want to relieve symptoms with drugs. Parents also want us to treat, to allay their fears, to comfort their children, at least to make them feel that they are doing something of use in a situation that frightens them and makes them feel helpless. Reaching for the prescription pad is such a reflex action for doctors that it may take an act of will to stop it. At the least, I think we should consider the effects and the meanings of our use of medicine.

The relationship of patients and doctors is profoundly and inevitably unequal. The patient comes needing help, wanting information, often fearing what has happened and what may be to come. The physician's place is one of the power of knowledge and the easy objectivity of distance, or so it appears to the patient. For the patient there is a tendency to regress to dependency, and often this engenders the angry resentment that can accompany a dependent state. For an independent adult or for an adolescent seeking independence, the classic physician-patient relationship is an uncomfortable mixture of fear, hope, grudging and partial trust, denial, and avoidance. For the doctor, the one-up position is ego-building, and we have a great many overbuilt egos to show for it. It also puts us on a pedestal from which we are very likely to fall (or be pushed). Not infrequently, we may find ourselves fighting resistance caused by this disequilibrium of power.

The relationship of these ideas to the use of medicine is that one can offer medicine as an option, instead of pushing medicine as an order. I think that there is a significant difference between saying "Give 120 mg of acetaminophen every 4 hours for fever" and saying "Now, if her fever seems to be making her uncomfortable, you might want to consider bringing it down with acetaminophen" and writing out the suggested dose. The difference is in the recognition, expressed in the choice of words, that the parent or the patient has the right to make decisions about treatment. For a broad range of children's illness, these choices do exist. Should symptoms be treated for the comfort of the patient or his family? Should a treatable disease be allowed to proceed without medical intervention because of a family's resistance to drug therapy? From time to time this question brings a family into court because of a life-threatening illness. In my practice the wisdom of intervening in everyday illness is questioned by parents week in and week out. A few years ago I gave a speech about the changing family to a local medical staff. During the discussion period an experienced pediatrician took the floor to denounce my permissiveness; failure to accept medical advice and treatment for a strep throat was child abuse in her book, and I should be ashamed of myself for countenancing it. Well, perhaps so, but if I see myself as a consultant rather than a cop, I'll do better to try to convince rather than convict. *Doctor,* after all, comes from the latin word *docere,* "to teach."

Tactics of Drug Use

A wise professor taught me that I should taste every medicine I prescribed in order to understand what I was asking my patients to endure. A useful extension of this advice is to imagine what it is like to take (or administer) the medicine every 6 hours around the clock.

Grossman's Laws of Drug Administration are as follows:

1. **Medicines should be prescribed to be taken as infrequently as possible.** A safe assumption is that daily or twice-daily dosing has a reasonable chance of success, at least as long as symptoms are troublesome. Dosing t.i.d. will be carried out at least half of the time. Dosing q.i.d. is a fantasy, except in the occasional family ruled by a parent with obsessive-compulsive disorder.

2. **Medicines should be taken at the most convenient times; this usually means at mealtimes, upon arising, or at bedtime.** Medicines prescribed at any other times will be forgotten. Multiple medications given on different dosing schedules will be confused initially and forgotten later.

3. **Find the formulation that is easiest to take.** Concentrated medicines mean less volume to struggle over. Chewable tablets don't spill from the spoon or dribble down the cheek. If a medicine tastes terrible, don't prescribe it if you can use something else. If you have to prescribe it, suggest ways to mask it with chocolate syrup or applesauce. Remember that different brands of the same drug may differ significantly in taste.

4. **Instruct the druggist to dispense the medicine in as many bottles as there are places where the child will be given the stuff.** A split family with two households needs two bottles; the day-care lady also may need a bottle.

5. **Teach little kids to take tablets as soon as possible.** The following methods are often helpful in teaching children over the age of 4 years to take tablets.

    a. Take a sip of water and hold it in your mouth; don't swallow it yet! Tilt your head back as far as you can. Toss a small, smooth, tablet-shaped candy into the puddle of water in the back of your mouth, and swallow. If this doesn't work the first time, eat the candy and try again.

b. Fill a clean, small-mouthed soda-pop or beer bottle with cold water. Place a small, smooth, tablet-shaped candy on your tongue. Drink rapidly from the bottle; the tablet will be washed down by the water.

6. **Don't neglect the rectum!** It is nearly impossible to coerce some kids into taking oral medicines. One can resort to the common European custom of rectal administration. It is certainly true that you may find yourself doing this in the absence of reliable data on rectal absorption, but it may be the only method available. A few medicines are ready-made in suppository form; others can be prepared, although the requests come their way so rarely that many pharmacists react with shock and disbelief at the notion. One can also have tableted medicines ground up and put into gelatin capsules. The parent pierces the capsule with a pin to speed dissolution and inserts it like a suppository.

7. **Generic medicines do not always equal the expensive, brand-name original.** This is sad but true, and one needs to be aware that treatment failures can result from an improperly formulated substitute.

8. **Write down your instructions to the family.** Nobody should be expected to remember medical instructions, because nobody will. Between the anxiety generated by the illness and the confusion of trying to understand medical jargon, parents are in no condition to retain what you tell them about their child's illness and its treatment. Speak simply and write legibly, and your patients will find a place for you in the local medical pantheon.

9. **When a treatment fails, consider the possibility that it was not used.** The innocent question "Did you have any trouble giving the medicine?" may reveal that it was never or hardly ever offered to the child. Maybe Great Aunt Sophie was thought to have reacted badly to a medicine that sounded similar to it, or dad preferred the homeopathic pills, or the bottle got spilled on the second day, or the kid just spit it out. There are lots of possibilities that the family will not necessarily volunteer information about because it is too embarrassing.

❦ CHAPTER 20

Allergic Disease

Allergy is a messy subject. Although the nonmedical world long ago decided that allergies account for most of the nonspecific misery of everyday life, our profession has never seemed to take allergy to its bosom. Like psychiatry, allergy is treated as the trouble-making and vaguely embarrassing poor relation of scientific medicine. In part this seems to be due to the faddish and cultish nonsense that clings to the field; a kind of Gresham's law obtains. The sad result is that many practitioners are poorly informed about allergy, and consequently a significant amount of allergic disease is neither diagnosed nor treated. This chapter touches briefly on some of the common allergic conditions that children bring to our offices; *asthma* is dealt with in Chapter 25 on chest disorders; *eczema* and *contact dermatitis* are discussed in Chapter 17 on skin diseases; and *allergic conjunctivitis* is included in Chapter 21 on eye problems.

Diagnosis, as always, starts with the history. The chronic stuffy nose that is worse overnight and upon arising suggests house dust mite or other household inhalant allergy. The seasonal coryza suggests pollens. The temporal relationship between a particular food and bizarre behavior turns one's attention to allergic fatigue-tension syndrome. Physical exam will help if the patient obliges you by showing dark-circled eyes; a pale, wet, and swollen nasal mucosa; a horizontal skin crease across the nose (from chronic nose-rubbing); or typical eczema. The lab can help by showing blood or nasal eosinophilia, or an elevated immunoglobulin E level. Specific antibodies to scores of allergens can be sought with the radioallergosorbent test (RAST). Many allergists claim that RASTs are less sensitive than skin testing,

205

but the advantages of the serologic tests are many. One can look for a vast array of suspected allergens without subjecting the child to repeated skin testing sessions. Skin testing, especially before the age of 3 or 4 years, is a difficult undertaking requiring a patient parent, a calm and quiet child, and a skillful skin tester. A set of 15 or 20 scratch tests takes a good hour in the office and is no great joy for any of the participants. A further advantage of the RAST is that a fully array of unstable skin test antigens need not be kept in one's office; in my experience the crucial antigen is always out of date and back-ordered at the supplier. It does seem to be the case that reproducibility of RAST and other similar tests varies, depending on the lab. I follow the advice of my friendly neighborhood allergist and use the RAST lab that she recommends.

If you decide to do skin scratch tests you will need extracts of the common pollens in your area; this will include trees, grasses, and weeds. Some labs will make up mixtures of pollens to decrease the number of scratches required, but this dilutes the individual antigens. Other antigens needed include molds, cat and dog dander and hair, house dust mite, cockroach (if they are common in your area), and perhaps some common foods. I have been unimpressed with the relationship between food skin tests and the patient's problems, but allergists swear by them. Histamine is used as a positive control. There are available devices that allow you to place eight antigens at a time with reasonable ease and in equivalent amounts. Make sure that the patient has had no antihistamine medication for at least a day before the test. Keep epinephrine close at hand in the room with the patient. If all this seems daunting, use RASTs instead and refer the undiagnosed remainder of your allergy patients to an allergist. An additional diagnostic tool is the elimination (Rowe) diet, which often helps to clarify the role of foods as allergens; a simplified version can be found in the discussion of eczema in Chapter 17.

Allergic Rhinitis

It is no surprise that inhalant allergens are the major causes of allergic nose problems; after all, that is where inhalants land in the greatest concentration. As mentioned, the history helps point to the probable causes. Time of year, climatic factors such as mold blooms in some areas, time of day, concomitant activities like house-cleaning or visits to dusty or cat hair–covered rooms—all these hints help to identify the cause. If the cause is a food allergy, it is likely to be something eaten frequently, like milk, wheat, or chocolate, so there may not be an obvious temporal relationship. If the nasal smear shows only polys and bacteria, this may be a bacterial infection superimposed on the allergy. Treat the infection vigorously and repeat the nasal smear if symptoms persist.

Treatment depends on etiology. Brief bouts of seasonal allergic rhinitis can often be handled with oral antihistamines. Long-acting and nonsedating terfenadine is excellent; the less costly chlorphenira-mine or brompheniramine, preferably in a sustained-action form, is often more sedating. Cromolyn nasal spray works well only if the child uses it often enough—2 or 3 times a day at least. Beclomethasone aqueous nasal spray or other local steroids are the most effective agents. Use the smallest dose possible for as short a period as you can; we do not know their long-term effects on children's noses. Keeping the child's room shut as much as possible and using an electronic air cleaner can be helpful as well. The availability of powerful drugs means that intractable hay fever is now a rarity, but some cases are so bad that hyposensitization shots are indicated.

Chronic allergic rhinitis is most often due to house dust mites, animal hair, and, in some areas, cockroaches; less frequent causes are household molds and foods. Avoidance and elimination are certainly preferred to chronic medication. Decreasing the house dust mite burden, even in a single room, is a remarkably difficult task. The mites live in rugs, upholstery, draperies, bed clothes, mattresses and box springs, and between floorboards. The room must be kept stripped bare and damp-mopped; the mattresses, box springs, and pillows must be encased in sealed plastic enclosures; and the bed covers must be washed in hot water every week or two. If the house has forced air heating, the vents should be sealed. Acaricides and mite antigen denaturing chemicals are now being used, but their efficacy is unknown.

Central Nervous System Allergy

A certain number of children in your practice will be miserable, edgy, complaining, fidgety, and perhaps hyperactive. Some of these kids will also have rather ordinary signs of respiratory or other organ system allergy. Before deciding that they need psychotherapy, methylpheni-date, or a different set of parents, it pays to consider the rare but real diagnosis of allergic tension fatigue syndrome. Aside from the likelihood that affected children have concomitant or previous allergic diseases, there are no good diagnostic clues to this condition, which appears to be a central nervous system allergy. Children with allergic tension fatigue syndrome differ from the patients with chronic fatigue syndrome in the absence of a precipitating illness. The usual cause is food allergy, typically wheat, cow's milk, or chocolate; a very few children react to food colors and artificial flavorings. Careful history-taking and an elimination diet will make the diagnosis. The patients I've followed have lost their food sensitivity slowly, over many years.

Urticaria

Aside from eczema, which is discussed in Chapter 17, urticaria is the most common allergic manifestation in the skin. Unfortunately for simplicity, urticarial rashes may have causes quite different from ordi-nary allergens. Cold urticaria, for example, looks and feels like any other case of hives, but it is a reaction to abrupt chilling, usually due to a cold swim. Cholinergic urticaria, on the other hand, results from overheating. In my experience, the most common cause of acute urti-caria is an oncoming systemic infection, usually a quite unimpressive viral syndrome. Papular urticaria as a reaction to insect bites is easily diagnosed, because the urticarial papules can be differentiated from the bites among which they are interspersed. When acute urticaria is due to a food or a medicine, the history is diagnostic. These rashes fade when the offending agent is avoided. One is left with a substantial group of urticarias without obvious cause; unhappily, these often per-sist or recur. Look for underlying systemic illness or hereditary angio-neurotic edema; when all your investigations are negative, look again at foods and medicines. Meanwhile, treat the child with antihistamines such as hydroxyzine, diphenhydramine, or cyproheptadine; you may need to try several drugs. Systemic steroids are a last resort.

Gastrointestinal Allergy

In infancy gastrointestinal reactions to foods are a dime a dozen. Colic can be caused by a variety of substances in breast milk, as well as by cow's milk or soy-based formulas. The colicky baby may manifest only discomfort, but there may also be vomiting or diarrhea, sometimes with blood; constipation is a much less common symptom of food allergy in infancy. The older infant is less likely to have gastrointestinal reactions to allergens; for some reason, the skin becomes the shock organ of choice, and eczema appears. However, some kids continue to have gastrointestinal allergies for years; any of these symptoms may be triggered by foods, or the child may just complain of belly pain within minutes or hours after an offending meal. Of course, severe food allergies may also trigger systemic reactions, including laryngospasm, bronchospasm, and anaphylaxis.

Nonallergic mechanisms can also be involved in adverse gastrointestinal reactions to foods. Inability to digest the lactose in milk is a common cause of pain, gas, and diarrhea. The incidence increases in later childhood, and the condition is most common among blacks and Asians, but anyone can be lactose-intolerant at any age. It is interesting that the degree of lactose intolerance can vary from time to time for no apparent reason. A few years ago much was written about lactose intolerance secondary to infectious gastroenteritis. Low-lactose formulas were advocated for use during and after the illness. The pendulum has now swung, and this much overdone fad has almost disappeared. Diarrhea is sometimes an overload reaction when an excess of food is consumed; I have seen this most often with starches. Constipation can occur in infancy when solids are first offered and the gastrointestinal tract is overwhelmed by its new task of digesting complex carbohydrates.

Allergy remains something of an enigma. Like syphilis or the Epstein-Barr virus, allergy can be a great imitator, hard to pin down, often a possible cause of disease, and always something to be kept in mind.

CHAPTER 21

Eye Problems

Our first task concerning the newborn baby's eyes is to check for abnormalities of structure and function. This is initially a straightforward procedure, once we get a good look past the tightly closed lids. In the first few weeks the baby should develop conjugate gaze, at least most of the time. The consequent development of tracking tells us about eye and cortical function. Later, we will be interested in testing binocular vision as early as possible. Unfortunately, there is no easy and reliable method of finding every amblyopic eye in the first years. Cover-uncover tests can be used late in the first year to assess fixation and reveal strabismus. An older infant can usually be induced to watch and follow a finger puppet as a target. Presenting a small, attractive toy on the floor or table near the a baby and watching for her apparent depth perception can give some additional information. The amblyopic baby can also be observed to become restless and unhappy when the better eye is covered. Anisometropia should be searched for by focusing the ophthalmoscope rapidly on each fundus; a difference of more than a few diopters is unusual. With luck, I find this can be done at about 1 year of age. By age 3 most children can be tested with what we term the "fly test," a simple device that shows apparent three-dimensionality; the manufacturers call it the Titmus Stereo Test (Titmus Optical Co., Petersburg, VA 23802). The more complex vision testing machines can be mastered by most 4-year-olds. If all this sounds like a lot of work, it is; the salvaging of an eye makes it worthwhile.

Conjunctivitis

At every-age the differential diagnosis of weepy eyes is a problem. During the newborn period we worry most about destructive gonococcal infections. Much more common are the low-grade mucopurulent discharges that start as early as the second day of life. A few of these turn out to be chlamydial infections, although these are most likely to appear later in the first week of life. When you see a well-developed chlamydial conjunctivitis with the characteristic intense redness and swelling of the palpebral conjunctiva, the diagnosis is fairly obvious. However, at the outset the signs can look unimpressive. Fortunately, for most of these first weeks of life, pussy eyes are caused by brief inflammations, bacteriologically unimpressive, and easily treated with sulfonamide or triple-antibiotic eye drops. If the discharge does not clear, keep in mind the possibility of congenital glaucoma as a cause of watery or mucoid tearing. The usual problem in chronic eye discharge in infancy is stenosis of the nasolacrimal duct. Massage to help open the duct is often recommended and occasionally carried out by especially compulsive parents; if there is any evidence that massage is useful, I'd like to see it. Antibiotic eye drops are needed to control the infection. Sometimes a single treatment a day is suppressive. Eventually, the vast majority of nasolacrimal ducts open up; if the eye is still wet and tearing at age 9 to 12 months, probing by your favorite ophthalmologist is in order.

In later childhood the differential diagnosis of conjunctivitis includes bacterial, viral, and allergic causes. The various infectious agents can produce similar clinical pictures: redness of the bulbar conjunctiva, especially peripherally; redness of the palpebral conjunctiva as well; itchy discomfort rather than the pain of uveitis; occasional photophobia; a mucoid or purulent discharge. Bacterial cases often accompany otitis (most often caused by *Haemophilus influenzae*), sinusitis, or ordinary common colds. Viral cases can look just about the same; the association of pharyngitis and conjunctivitis caused by the adenovirus may be distinctive. In allergic cases the conjunctiva is often bumpy or cobbled in appearance, and the bulbar conjunctiva may have a swollen, raw-egg-white appearance. The discharge is usually watery or mucoid rather than frankly purulent; itching is intense, and other signs of inhalant allergy may be present in the nose and chest.

One ends up either treating for allergy or using an antibiotic (locally or systemically) for a presumed bacterial cause. Allergic conjunctivitis does not generally respond to oral antihistamines, even when they control other allergic symptoms. Topical antihistamine and decongestant combinations (pheniramine or pyrilamine with naphazoline or phenylephrine) work well, but they sting; cromolyn 4% takes a day or two to help but is then quite effective; and weak steroids (prednisolone 0.12% suspension) are excellent as a last resort. Systemic antibiotic treatment for conjunctivitis is justified if there is a coexisting sinusitis or otitis. Sometimes systemic treatment is necessary just because it is so difficult to get adequate amounts of local medication onto the eyes. For treating small children, drops are easier to use than ointment. One trick is to have the child lie supine with eyes closed. Several drops are placed at the inner corner of the child's closed lids. When the eyes are opened, the drops flood in without much discomfort. Eye ointment has the advantage of persistence; you can probably get away with fewer daily doses. The lower lid should be pulled down and everted and a ribbon of ointment laid from one corner to the other, between lid and bulb. The eye should then be held open for about 30 seconds to allow the ointment to melt and spread. If you fail to tell the parents how to apply these medications, they will be used imaginatively but not effectively.

Sunburn Conjunctivitis

This is a disorder of affluence. It is seen in skiers during the springtime when the bright sun bounces off the snow, and in boaters who fail to wear sunglasses. It really hurts. The eyes are bright red, the lids are swollen and there is usually a nice sunburn of the skin as well. Use aspirin or a nonsteroidal anti-inflammatory agent by mouth and weak steroid eye drops like prednisolone suspension 0.12%.

Cellulitis, Orbital and Periorbital (Preseptal)

Orbital cellulitis is not a topic for a book on everyday pediatrics; it is obviously a severe condition treated in the hospital by pediatrician and ophthalmologist together. I mention it only to contrast it with the much more manageable periorbital or preseptal cellulitis. Usually one makes the differentiation easily. In periorbital infection the eye moves well, there is no pain in the eye itself, there is no proptosis, and vision is normal. The redness and swelling of the lids often extend down to the cheek, and a violaceous hue is common. The patient is likely to be a toddler or a young child. The patient with orbital cellulitis is usually older and has a painful and swollen eye that moves poorly. If you are not sure which entity is in front of you, a computed tomographic scan and an ophthalmologist will be a great help. If the case is a straightforward periorbital cellulitis, consider outpatient treatment with ceftriaxone given intramuscularly or amoxicillin-clavulanate or cefuroxime axetil given orally. Daily follow-up visits, reliable phone communications, and stable parents are essential.

Corneal Abrasion

To treat the child with corneal abrasion, start by instilling a drop of local anesthetic solution (proparacaine or tetracaine), then put another drop at the end of a strip of fluorescein paper. Touch the wet end to the conjunctiva, and have the child close the eye. This method minimizes discomfort and uses the least amount of fluorescein, so you don't have to spend so much effort washing away the extra dye. If there is no sign of a foreign body, further treatment is purely for symptoms; corneal scrapes heal rapidly without any help. However, it is a good idea to instill a blob of antibiotic ophthalmic ointment and then place an occlusive patch. The eye needs protection from being rubbed during the 15 minutes or so for which the local anesthesia lasts. When it wears off, the photophobia and pain will return if the eye is not patched, at least for a few hours. Rechecking the corneal abrasion the next day will ensure that you have not overlooked a foreign body. The eye will nearly always feel and look fine in a day. A fluorescein exam is rarely needed at that time.

❦ CHAPTER 22

Gastrointestinal Disorders

It appears that every culture focuses attention on its favorite organ system. The Germans worry about circulatory failure and low blood pressure; the French are concerned about the state of their livers; American parents worry about the gastrointestinal tract, especially its intake and output. In the foregoing chapters we have already looked at food and constipation. Now we address vomiting, diarrhea, and the other more common problems of the gut.

Gastroesophageal Reflux

Is gastroesophageal reflux really a common problem? The difficulty in thinking about reflux is that spitting up stomach contents is an absolutely normal infant activity. Nearly every baby spits up, most of them quite frequently. After a few months of age spitting up may diminish, but it worsens later in the first year when the infant starts to creep and crawl; a vigorous infant in the prone position can push a lot of food out of his stomach. There is a considerable decrease in regurgitation in the toddler years, but at any age a certain amount of reflux happens. Usually the only result is a temporary bad taste in the mouth. Esophagitis, aspiration pneumonia, and recurrent asthma can develop as a result of frequent and copious gastroesophageal reflux, but they should not be our first thought every time we see a 2-year-old spit up. The trap here is hidden in the questions of when and how to evaluate the spitter, and what significance to give to the findings. A high-tech study may demonstrate regurgitation, but it does not prove

215

a causal relationship to the child's other symptoms. Both the tests (which are multiple) and the treatments (which are not very effective) are currently in flux; the clinician should take all recommendations with a good dose of salt.

Vomiting

The clinician who takes care of children learns quickly to be wary about vomiting. This is true in several ways. First, one learns to move very rapidly out of range of a retching child; a vomitus-coated shirt front can ruin your whole day. Second, vomiting is one of those symptoms, like wheezing, that usually have an unexciting and straightforward etiology but that once in a while are caused by something wholly unexpected. One could fill a page with lists of diseases that start out with emesis. Third, the significance of vomiting depends on the child's age. Real vomiting in infancy, not just spitting up, is always important. Fourth, every child has favorite symptoms; some kids vomit with every little illness, but other kids vomit hardly at all. When one of the latter group throws up, pay attention.

Management of the vomiting associated with the common nongastrointestinal diseases of childhood does not usually amount to much. When a child vomits because she is coming down with a strep throat or a kidney infection or because she has asthma or a dozen other nongastrointestinal diseases, the throwing up is usually early in the illness and it rarely needs to be treated. If the vomiting persists, a few doses on an antiemetic may be needed, especially if the child is to be given oral medication for the underlying acute disease. The most powerful antiemetics are phenothiazines, among which chlorpromazine is an excellent choice. The syrup is absorbed so quickly that it usually stops vomiting in one or two doses. Rectal suppositories are also available. Don't use prochlorperazine; the incidence of quite frightening extrapyramidal symptoms is too high in children. Trimethobenzamide (Tigan) and promethazine (Phenergan) are heavily promoted as antiemetics, but they don't work very well.

In treating vomiting from any acute illness, gastrointestinal or otherwise, for decades it has been customary to limit oral intake to clear liquids with a gradual resumption of dilute milk and then light solids. Recently a number of studies have purported to prove that much more aggressive feeding regimens are superior. There is no doubt that total weight loss can be minimized by giving foods of higher caloric density from the beginning. This is probably of some importance when the patient is chronically malnourished at the outset. However, for the usual American child the old standard regimen is decidedly easier and it works very well.

The sick child is most likely to accept clear sweet liquids during the first day of illness, and he is certainly less likely to vomit if he is given only small amounts at frequent intervals. The choice of liquids has been exhaustively studied, and practitioners have been scolded for our loyalty to the wrong, old solutions. What seems not be have been noted is that the wrong, old solutions are successful; they are easily available, taste pretty good, and don't cost much. I usually use the commercially available electrolyte solutions if the patient is a small infant or if a considerable degree of dehydration has already occurred. Otherwise, I ask parents to use a variety of clear liquids, including apple juice, any kind of soda pop that is not sugar-free, Gatorade, weak tea with sugar, Jello water (Jello made with twice the usual amount of water so that it will not gel), and frozen fruit juice bars. Rice water, the supernatant liquid obtained by boiling rice, is another excellent first liquid. Start with 5 to 15 ml every 10 minutes for about an hour, and then slowly increase the volume over the next few hours. As the child takes larger amounts he may want the liquids somewhat less frequently. When the vomiting has subsided I ask them to alternate clear chicken broth (as a source of Na^+ and K^+) and a sweet liquid.

Sometimes improvement is so rapid that bland solids and milk can be given on the first day; more often one waits until the second day. The choice of solids depends on the illness. If there is no associated diarrhea, it is unlikely to matter what solids the child eats once the vomiting has stopped. If diarrhea is present, you can usually count on making it worse with coarse, high-residue, and spicy foods. A "white" diet of milk, noddles, white rice, white bread and white cereal, banana, apple, and potato is usually acceptable. It may take several days before a child can digest a normal diet without cramps and more loose stools. An interesting exception in the management of vomiting is the breast-fed infant. These babies often keep down small, frequent nursings, although they would vomit more generous breast feeds. Often it is possible to give small amounts of clear fluids alternated with brief nursings from the outset of the illness.

Diarrhea

Unlike vomiting, which is a strikingly nonspecific symptom in childhood, diarrhea is much more likely to signify true gastrointestinal disease. Of course, a modest amount of diarrhea can be part of many nongastrointestinal illnesses, but it will rarely amount to anything important and can often be ignored.

Academic discussions of diarrhea make the important distinction between acute and chronic symptoms. Unfortunately for the patient and the practitioner, the onsets of these two quite different problems are typically identical, namely, loose stools. It would help if the patients came with prognostic labels, but since this is unusual, we all tend to expect that the child with a new case of diarrhea has one of the common viral gastroenteritis infections. Of course, we abandon that assumption if there is high fever, blood in the stool, jaundice, hepatomegaly, or other signs of more dramatic disease. Ordinarily, the child with acute diarrhea is not terribly sick. If he does have one of the many viral gastrointestinal infections, he has probably started with vomiting and malaise and a slight fever. He complains of cramps and has no appetite. There may be a family or community outbreak of similar illnesses. Physical findings are usually limited to signs of an overactive gut. The prudent physician prescribes a limited diet along the lines of the antivomiting regimen already described, and arranges to stay in touch with the family. Antidiarrheal drugs are unlikely to be needed and carry a small risk; if this turns out to be a significant bacterial gastrointestinal infection, you do not want to paralyze the gut. This is a low-tech approach: no lab tests, no drugs, just proper fluids and a little patience.

When the illness is more severe or otherwise atypical of viral gastrointestinal infection, you will need help from the lab. An excellent and often neglected test is a smear of stool (or stool mucus) for polys. The correlation with bacterial infection is high enough to be a guide to further studies. The usual stool cultures and ova and parasite exams pose a variety of problems. They are terribly costly and prone to error. A single stool culture sometimes misses a significant pathogen, and O and P exams are so often falsely negative that we have all been taught to take at least three samples. In the case of *Giardia* infections, the *Giardia* antigen test is decidedly more sensitive and should be used if that is what you are looking for. The presence of a variety of organisms of questionable pathogenicity is another dilemma. What do we do when the stool is found to contain *Cryptosporidium, Isospora,* or *Blastocystis?* Although these organisms are not likely to cause symptoms in immunocompetent hosts, it is tempting to treat them if the child is very sick. The unproven effectiveness of antibiotics in these cases is a further deterrent to intervention.

When diarrhea persists, one begins to consider a rather different set of causes, including food allergy, inflammatory bowel disease, and malabsorption problems. One syndrome that causes more trouble than it is worth is the "normal" diarrhea that can occur in perfectly healthy older infants and toddlers. These are typically big, happy, vigorous kids with big appetites; they grow normally and have little or no sign of discomfort, but their stools are large, wet, and frequent. All the appropriate tests come back normal and the parents begin to wonder about seeing a gastroenterologist. His tests come back normal, too. After a number of months the diarrhea subsides. Because the etiology is wholly unknown, treatment is empiric, to say the least. Sometimes the problem seems to be an overload of a particular group of foods; sometimes it is related to an excessively low-fat diet. Experimentation with diet is about the most one can offer.

Some episodes of diarrhea are sufficiently severe or prolonged that drug treatment is worth trying. Bismuth subsalicylate (Pepto-Bismol) is known to be useful against "turista," and it sometimes works with domestic diarrheas as well. The amount of absorbed salicylate should be considered but doesn't really seem to be a problem. Cholestyramine is a resin that helps diarrhea by binding a variety of irritants within the gut. It has been used alone in doses of one fourth to one half of a 9-gm packet 2 to 4 times a day. Because it is a gritty powder, kids resist it; try mixing it with a small volume of apple juice. One South African study showed a good effect when cholestyramine was given with oral gentamicin; the drugs were given 1 hour apart to minimize binding of the gentamicin.

Recurrent Abdominal Pain

Am I the only one, or do all physicians have favorite diseases? In order for a disease to be truly enjoyable from the point of view of the practitioner, it has to have certain clear-cut characteristics. These include (1) relative rarity so that the diagnosis is intellectually satisfying, (2) the possibility of a precise diagnosis that cannot be gainsaid, and (3) a benign, nonfatal course. Recurrent abdominal pain does meet criterion #3, but it is absolutely nobody's favorite disease. Whose heart has not sunk at the first description of intermittent, variable, hard-to-describe bellyache? The patient is most often a middle-aged child, usually a girl, who looks sad but not particularly unhealthy. The physical exam findings are negative; the pain is more or less periumbilical. The doctor's dilemma is diagnostic. In one's heart of hearts, one knows that there is no demonstrable physical problem to be found, but a certain minimum number of investigations are required. A complete blood count, urinalysis, and urine culture will reassure everyone. Fancier studies, especially radiography or ultrasound, should be avoided if possible. The more studies that are done, no matter how negative the results, the more everyone is taught the message "There is a disease at the root of this, which must be found!" What is truly at the root of these pains is likely to be emotional tension, probably evidencing itself in some kind of intestinal motility response. In adult medicine this is termed "irritable bowel syndrome," and large quantities of antispasmodics and tranquilizers are thrown at it. This therapeutic approach seems quite wrong for children. I think we do much better to listen to the complaint, lean back, and say that pains like these are usually a sign of anxiety or tension or emotional struggle in a child's life. Therefore, the way to manage it is to invest some time and effort in figuring out what the problems might be. Schedule one or two half-hour talk visits over the next week, seeing the parents separately from the child, if you can. Get some information about what is happening in the family and at school. Try to avoid reaching for the prescription pad; home remedies like a hot bath or warm milk or generic tender loving care may be sufficient. Sometimes the symptom disappears as soon as the child realizes that someone cares about her troubles. More often it waxes and wanes for no clear reason. After a visit or two with the child and her parents, a psychological etiology may have become obvious enough to everyone so that a referral to a psychotherapist will be accepted. Not infrequently, the talk visits are sufficiently clarifying and therapeutic that nothing else is required.

The problem with this approach to bellyache is that it is opposite to the way we ordinarily proceed. We have all been taught to "rule out" organic disease at all costs, even when a complaint is 99% likely to be psychosomatic. We are all terrified of missing a zebra in a herd of horses. Fortunately, the only organic problems that require prompt treatment are urinary tract disorders, which are nearly always found with a urinalysis and culture. Other organic problems, such as peptic ulcer and inflammatory bowel disease, can look unimportant at the outset. However, they soon enough make their presence known with increasing and diverse symptoms. In short, with the usual case of recurrent abdominal pain one has the luxury of proceeding deliberately, focusing on the likely diagnosis first. If emotional factors are not uncovered by a few office interviews, one can go on to consider food intolerance, lactase deficiency, celiac syndrome, gastritis, ulcers, *Giardia*, other parasites, and inflammatory bowel disease.

❧ CHAPTER 23

Genitourinary Disorders

Urinary Tract Infections

"UTI" is a misleading acronym that needs to be discarded. The various infections of the kidneys, bladder, and urethra subsumed are so different in etiology and management that one cannot and should not think of them as a clinical entity. It would make as much sense as bundling the common cold and lobar pneumonia into one category.

Pyelonephritis

The differences between academic and practice approaches to disease are well-illustrated by kidney infections. The textbook teaches that bag urines are unreliable; the practitioner finds that bag urines carefully collected in the home or office are usually sufficient, especially if multiple samples are consistent. The hospital-based physician is likely to treat the child with pyelonephritis in the hospital by using parenteral antibiotics. The office-based practitioner has discovered that his patients do quite well with oral antibiotics given at home.

The diagnosis of pyelonephritis is usually straightforward, once it occurs to us to look for it. Until the patient is old enough to report flank pain, we must consider somewhat more subtle clues. Prolonged jaundice in the newborn, unexplained vomiting with fever in the older child, repeated episodes of fever, and malaise at any age: any of these can suggest kidney infection. Pyuria or urine dipsticks positive for leukocyte esterase or nitrite will indicate a urine culture. The standard

50,000 colonies/ml as evidence of a significant level of bacteriuria is misleadingly high. When you collect clean-catch or bag urine specimens in the office setting, you will often find fewer organisms, probably because the cultures are set up promptly. A colony count as low as 10,000/ml is likely to signify urinary tract infection, especially if it is a pure culture. A second specimen is useful to confirm infection, but one will not always choose to wait to obtain it.

In our practice we have found it laborious but possible to get the information we need with voided urines in nearly all instances. At any age the first requirement is a well-cleaned genital and perineal area. Foreskins need to be retracted as much as possible, vulvas need thorough soap and water washing, vaginal secretions need to be rinsed away. This will be done effectively only if the parent, patient, or nurse knows precisely what is needed. In infants, the use of a plastic urine collection bag will succeed only if the area is clean and the surrounding skin is dry, and if the bag is removed promptly after the child urinates. It is always necessary to show the parent exactly how the collection bag is to be applied, if the specimen is to be collected at home. The application of a bag at bedtime with an attempt at retrieval the next morning is a complete waste of time. For the toilet-trained girl we have often used a cleverly designed potty chair that holds a sterile cup below and in front of the child's urethra. As she begins to void, the initial portion of the urine falls into the pot, and as her stream velocity increases, the stream moves anteriorly into the sterile cup, yielding an automatic midstream specimen. When it works, it's great.

Very rarely, you will not be able to obtain a convincing urine sample by bag or clean catch. My own preference is to catheterize the patient, rather than do a bladder puncture. We use an infant feeding tube (8-French size) as the catheter; it is sterile, disposable, and so smooth that it doesn't hurt.

The role of radiographic, radionuclide, and sonographic studies in the diagnosis and follow-up of pyelonephritis is a vexed question. In the last analysis, the diagnosis is clinical; short of a renal biopsy, there can be no single gold-standard test. A decidedly skeptical frame of mind is appropriate in evaluating each newly proposed method. In every case, one asks whether the information gained from a test will change one's management of this patient. Because so many little girls have only one episode of pyelonephritis, close follow-up with urinalyses and urine cultures may obviate the necessity for more invasive procedures. If the circumstances suggest that follow-up will be difficult to accomplish, it makes sense to obtain a sonogram, possibly a renal cortical scan, and a voiding cystourethrogram or radionuclide isocystogram when the child is well. Because of the higher incidence of demonstrable pathology in little boys, studies of the upper tract plus a voiding cystourethrogram should be done after the first episode of pyelonephritis.

Treatment will vary with the circumstances. The septic newborn with pyelonephritis will be in the hospital nursery and will probably get ampicillin and gentamicin. The newborn who is not all that ill may well have been discharged home; consider oral therapy with amoxicillin or a cephalosporin, depending on sensitivity tests. Remember to tell the lab you want sensitivities measured at urine, rather than serum, levels. Past infancy, you can use a sulfonamide such as sulfisoxazole or sulfamethoxazole. These agents have worked well for years; they are less likely to cause allergic reactions than trimethoprim-sulfamethoxazole. Amoxicillin is another good alternative. The oral cephalosporins are expensive but well-tolerated. An occasional resistant organism can be treated with nitrofurantoin; be sure to use the macrocrystals, not the tablets or suspension, which cause too much vomiting.

A follow-up urine culture on the third day of treatment should be sterile. I generally give 7 to 10 days of antibiotic, wait 2 to 3 days, and get another urine culture.

All these cultures cost the patient a fortune if they are done by hospital or commercial labs. Furthermore, you will never get the results promptly. With your own office lab, you can usually have results in less than a day, and costs can be kept down. We use one MacConkey agar plate and one blood agar plate, inoculate with a calibrated 0.01-ml loop, and set up sensitivities only as needed and only with drugs we are likely to use. Sometimes, we set up sensitivities directly from obviously infected urine without waiting for the culture; this shortcut does not always work, the usual problem being contamination with a spreading *Proteus*.

Cystitis

This is a mixed group. Sometimes you will see bladder infections for no apparent reason in children of any age. However, most of my patients with cystitis are sexually active adolescent girls, often, in fact, sexually overactive; the episodes follow a period of unusually frequent or enthusiastic intercourse. The dysuria, frequency, and little, if any, fever will point to a lower tract infection; the culture will nearly always show *Escherichia coli*. Improvement is much quicker than in the child with pyelonephritis. The same oral antibiotics can be given for 1 week or more; brief courses lead to frequent relapse. One important goal is relieving the discomfort with phenazopyridine; it works instantly. For children too young to take the tablets, ask the pharmacist to make up a syrup form. Warn the patient or parent that the urine will turn bright orange! This is very dramatic if not anticipated. The adolescents with postcoital cystitis tend to have recurrences. These can be fairly well controlled by a simple routine: (1) Drink a glass of water before intercourse. (2) Void and drink another glass of water after intercourse. Unfortunately, adolescents are not likely to follow simple routines. Some patients will get repeated bouts of infection, unless they take a single dose of a sulfonamide or nitrofurantoin before love-making.

The necessity for follow-up studies depends on age, sex, and circumstances. The rare instance of cystitis in a little boy requires a thorough radiologic and sonographic workup. A first episode of cystitis in a little girl merits follow-up urinalyses and cultures for at least 1 year, but further studies only if there are recurrences. The sexually active teenager with cystitis will rarely need any studies other than urinalyses and cultures.

Urethritis

The issue with urethritis is the extent and direction of associated disease. It can be difficult to discover whether the bladder is also involved, if the urethra is the only site, or if a local vulvitis is the real problem. Uncomplicated urethritis should express itself with dysuria, noted especially at the end of urination; sometimes there will be terminal hematuria or urethral discharge. Older children and adolescents can provide a "first glass" specimen from the beginning of urination, which will represent the urethra, and a "second glass" midstream specimen, which will largely reflect the state of the bladder. If there is only a little pyuria in the second specimen, it is often reasonable to treat the local symptoms overnight while awaiting urine culture results. Forced fluids, phenazopyridine by mouth, and sitz baths followed by the application of polysporin-bacitracin ointment; these usually control discomfort. Teenagers with urethritis may need cultures for *Chlamydia* and *Neisseria gonorrhoeae*; make no assumptions about virginity or its absence. Remember your own youth (or that of your friends) and how easy it was to dissemble about your degree of sexual experience. The trick is to ask the right questions and get honest answers; it helps to have the parent absent from the examining room.

Urethritis in small children is often irritative rather than infective. This is sometimes associated with vulvitis, but not always. The common cause is bubble bath; shampoo in the bath water is alleged to be another irritant, but I have never come across a case. Rarely, the etiology is dietary, usually an excess of orange juice. Once the child is bathing herself, she may successfully resist her parent's efforts to wash her genitals. This may lead to a chronic, mild vulvitis and urethritis. It is worth culturing for yeast and for bacteria, especially beta streptococcus. If the cultures are negative, treatment is simple. Have the child bathe daily, sitting with her thighs abducted, and tell the parents to insist on supervising the final washing and rinsing. After the bath, polysporin-bacitracin ointment should be applied. A week of this routine is usually enough.

Vulvitis and Vaginitis

When your patient is an adolescent, diagnosis and treatment of vulvitis and vaginitis are fairly straightforward. Sexually transmitted infections, candidiasis, *Gardnerella* (nonspecific) vaginitis, and foreign bodies are the major possibilities. Appropriate examination may not be easy, but it is usually possible, especially if the patient already has a trusting relationship with you. Because I include a visual exam of the external genitals in every full physical exam from infancy onward, the girls in my practice are generally fairly relaxed when they have their first complete pelvic exam. Because I want to avoid the message "Pelvics are a big deal!" the exam is usually done on a regular table, without drapes or stirrups or a chaperone. Even if the first pelvic exam is done during an episode of infection or inflammation, it can be reasonably comfortable for an unfrightened teenager. Regarding the prepubertal girl, a great deal has been written about allegedly specific anatomic evidence of sexual abuse. I think we need to approach this with much skepticism. Between the confounding problems of innocent injuries ("straddle" or otherwise induced) plus normal anatomic variability, the opportunities for clinical judgment to go awry are impressive. Any kind of internal exam is a problem with prepubertal kids. I know the experts want us to do intravaginal exams in little girls with vaginitis, but sometimes it can be avoided. Unless there is a bloody discharge, I settle for examining the external genitals and getting cultures from the vaginal orifice. I use cotton swabs moistened by rubbing them over the surfaces of the culture media: Biggy agar for yeast and blood agar for *Streptococcus*. You may also want to get a wet mount for *Trichomonas,* a smear for clue cells (for *Gardnerella*), and cultures for *N. gonorrhoeae* and *Chlamydia*. We use canine otoscope tips for the rare instance requiring a look into the vagina. If this can't be done, it may be necessary for a gynecologist to do the exam under a light anesthetic.

The most common vulvovaginal infection in little girls is candidiasis. Intravaginal topical treatment is difficult or impossible, but fortunately one can get by nicely with generous vulvar applications of antiyeast creams such as clotrimazole or miconazole. Candidiasis in adolescents may become a recurrent problem, which can usually be controlled by prolonged courses of treatment. If the patient has a pattern of yeast infection following the use of antibiotics, using a few prophylactic doses of clotrimazole or miconazole makes sense.

Vulvar Adhesions

The usual patient is a plump infant whose labia minora are held closely together by the surrounding fat rolls of thigh. Washing her bottom is so difficult that it isn't done often, and the moist mucosal surfaces begin to adhere posteriorly. If this is pointed out to the parents, they may be able to reverse the process with more diligent washing. If the adhesion increases anteriorly, covering the vaginal orifice and approaching the urethral meatus, it is probably worth treating. I say "probably" because I am not sure how much difficulty is actually caused by this little curtain of tissue; the urine always seems to find a way out. Furthermore, vaginal adhesions are very likely to disappear by midchildhood. If you decide to treat the child, applying a dab of estrogen cream (dienestrol, estradiol, or conjugated estrogens) b.i.d. for about 2 weeks usually suffices to separate the labia. However, recurrences are frequent. Excessive amounts of locally applied estrogen can cause temporary breast changes; be sparing.

❧ CHAPTER 24

Ear, Nose, and Throat Disorders

The clinician who treats children spends more time managing ear, nose, and throat problems than anything else. Efficient techniques of examination will make a considerable difference in what we find and how easily we find it. The most important skill you can have in ear, nose, and throat exams is mastery of the head mirror. This wonderful, low-tech device allows you to have two hands free and to have a bright light wherever you need it, including in ear canals, noses, throats, and, for a different group of problems, vaginas. It makes a significant difference in the retrieval of tiny foreign bodies stuck in the throat, for ear-cleaning, and for the management of epistaxis, to mention only a few situations.

Ear-cleaning is, of course, the bête noire of the pediatrician. Faced with a screaming kid, a parent who is unable to hold the child still, and a canal full of ear wax, who has not wanted to switch to radiology? If the ear wax is the hard, pebbly, or flaky variety that Chinese and Japanese children are particularly likely to have, or if the canal is tender and friable, there is a certain temptation to guess what is going on instead of thoroughly cleaning the canal and getting a good look. To remove wax you need a delicate cerumen spoon with smooth surfaces; Stortz makes a good one. You also need a rough-ended wire device on which you can twist a wisp of cotton for cleaning those ears too small for a standard cotton swab; an expensive but fairly adequate substitute is a ready-made nasopharyngeal swab. Sometimes it helps to moisten the swab with alcohol. Often you will need to soften ear wax. The best all-around solution is liquid dish detergent, 1 part in 20 parts tap water. Fill the canal with the dilute

231

detergent, plug it with some cotton, and return 15 minutes later to clean the nicely softened wax. We keep a dropper bottle of this in every examination room. If this fails, a proprietary surfactant called Cerumenex is effective. Unfortunately, it is irritating and must be washed out of the canal afterward, which makes it difficult to use in the presence of any infection. Carbamide peroxide is a much slower-acting cleanser; used once or twice a day for a few days before an exam, it usually leaves the canal in an easy-to-clean state. Yes, this is a lot of trouble, but you absolutely must see the tympanic membranes, especially if the child is ill.

The examination of the mouth and pharynx is often done by asking the patient to open wide, protrude the tongue, and say "Ah." This has two unfortunate consequences. The back of the tongue is brought forward where the tongue blade can touch it; this is likely to provoke retching and vomiting. It will also cause the pharynx to contract, thereby forcing the tonsils toward the midline and making them look bigger than they really are. The examiner, eager to avoid being vomited on, gets only a brief and misleading look while jumping back out of range. A better method is to ask the patient to open the mouth and pant; one must demonstrate this for small children, who are usually quite amused. Panting lets the tongue relax out of the way, the tongue blade touches only the front of the tongue, minimizing retching, and the tonsils can be seen in their normal position.

The Common Cold and Other Simple Upper Respiratory Infections

The treatment of trivial upper respiratory infections provides us with a useful opportunity to teach families how to think about diseases and therapies, including how and when to take temperatures, how to manage contagion, and when to call the doctor. Part of this teaching is done consciously and deliberately, as we provide information about the causes and likely course of an illness. At least as important is the nonverbal teaching we do, largely without our own awareness, by the manner and tenor of our own approach to disease. A tense and worried practitioner with an aggressive approach to the management of disease soon teaches patients to be tense and worried with every illness. If you rush in with lab studies and drug treatment for every upper respiratory infection, the lesson is that medical intervention is necessary, expected, and probably important. In short, a nervous doctor makes nervous patients.

Of course, your approach will reflect how you really feel, and this is not totally under your conscious control. However, it may be possible to cultivate a somewhat more stolid demeanor. You can be honest with parents about the likely diagnosis of an illness without providing them with a differential diagnosis of all the rare and fatal possibilities that cross your mind. You can even experiment with tone of voice and cadence of speech; there are calming ways of conveying information and there are tension-making ways. One of my families teases me that I always preface an answer with "Well now, . . ." in a fairly transparent attempt to keep everyone peaceful. Well now, it works with them.

The parents of a sick child will not remember much of what you tell them during an office visit or a phone conversation, but they will want a general idea about the likely cause and expected course of the illness. They need to know what complications to watch for, when to be in touch with you again, and what treatment is needed. We need to help parents understand the uses and limitations of therapy. Especially for self-limited and basically trivial diseases, people need to understand that the human body generally does a great job of getting over illness. If the proposed treatment is unduly vigorous, the underlying message is that you can't get over anything without a visit to the doctor and an expensive drug. This is not to say that we should ignore symptomatic therapy when there is something to offer. A few hours of nasal decongestion can be a considerable help at times, and so can a few hours of cough suppression. You will not shorten the duration of the cold, but the patient will have an easier time with it.

Temperature control is a particularly good area for helping parents understand illness. If they are taught that fever is an important defense mechanism rather than an enemy to be fought, they can be much more relaxed about childhood disease. When I am asked at what temperature to give an antipyretic, I usually say "104° or 105°F if she seems uncomfortable." The important message is that you really do not have to fight fever; give an antipyretic if the fever itself seems to trouble the child. A 2-year-old with roseola can be running around the house playing happily with a very high fever; she does not need medicine at all. On the other hand, a child can be achy and miserable at 100.5°F and benefit from aspirin or acetaminophen. The indication for the antipyretic is misery, not temperature elevation per se. What parents also need to know about fever is that the course of a fever gives some useful information about the development of the disease and sometimes hints at the duration of contagiousness. A reasonable rule of thumb is that the common illnesses of childhood can be considered to be contagious until the child is free of fever for 24 hours. I know that this is unscientific and inaccurate, but as approximations go, it is useful. It also underlines the fact that temperatures are lowest in the morning so that a child who is afebrile at 8:00 A.M. may still be sick and have recurrent fever a bit later in the day when the eager parent may have sent him off to school. Normal temperature should be below 99°F on arising and below 100°F later in the day.[1]

Most parents need to be taught how to take temperatures. They need to know that axillary temperatures are fairly accurate during early infancy but are quite untrustworthy later. I suppose this change is due to the insulating effect of the maturing skin. They also need to know that the colored fever strips applied to the forehead reveal a lot about skin temperature but not much about true, internal body temperature. I think they are a waste of time. Many parents convince themselves that the estimation of temperature by touch is sufficient. For this reason I always ask, "When did you last measure the child's temperature?" rather than, "Does she have a fever?" Answers to the latter question may simply reflect the custom of mother's lips or fingers briefly applied to child's forehead, a lovely gesture but not of much use.

Rectal temperature-taking tends to upset everyone, but this is the most accurate measure available. The rule of thumb that rectal is 1°F higher than oral is wrong; the metabolic activity of bacteria in the stool may sometimes increase the rectal temperature reading, but this is not a uniform phenomenon. When a standard glass thermometer is used, the mercury should be shaken down only to about 98°F; it will take a lot less time for an accurate reading to be made, and

[1] Mackowiak PA, Wasserman SS, Levine MM: A Critical Appraisal of 98.6°F. JAMA 1992; 268:1578–1580.

this is particularly appreciated when a rectal temperature is being taken. The baby or small child should be placed on the parent's lap, the buttocks spread and the thermometer gently inserted less than an inch into the anal canal. If the thermometer is rotated back and forth between the fingers as it is placed, a lubricant will not be needed and the whole process is simpler. When the thermometer is in place, use one hand braced against the buttocks and thighs to hold it steady and hold the child's back firmly with the other hand. About 1 minute is needed for the mercury to rise from 98°F to an accurate reading. Once parent and child learn that this is a painless and manageable procedure, temperature monitoring will be done with less resistance.

Having finally decided that the child has a common cold, what treatment options should you offer the family? Decongestant nose drops are a mistake. They paralyze ciliary cleansing of the nose and sinuses, and they cause rebound congestion. Salt and baking soda nose drops will help babies to breathe better for a brief time; this can make a nice difference when a baby is so stuffy that she can't nurse and breathe at the same time. Table salt, 1/4 teaspoon, and baking soda, 1/4 teaspoon, are added to 8 ounces of tap water; use several drops in each nostril as often as needed. A good way to instill them is with the baby supine on the parent's lap, her neck extended, and her head clamped between the parent's knees. Hold the flailing arms with one hand and use a medicine dropper to instill the salt and soda solution slowly into the nostrils. Unlike regular decongestant solutions, these drops do not sting; a fresh batch can be made up every day if needed.

Oral decongestants don't seem to do much for infants. In older kids, either pseudoephedrine or phenylpropanolamine, with or without an antihistamine, will provide some easier breathing. The syrups and the standard tablet forms usually work for a few hours. The long-acting granular preparations designed for adults can be used for kids; open a capsule and sprinkle one third or one half of the contents onto a little applesauce or ice cream. One problem with all these drugs is that they tend to interfere with normal ciliary motion. Phenylpropanolamine often decreases appetite and causes irritability; because sick kids are already anorexic and fussy, this approach seems truly egregious. Cough suppressants are sometimes quite useful. Codeine certainly works the best, but it is sedating and causes constipation and nausea. A few patients manifest an idiosyncratic reaction with vomiting and weakness; this may be due to codeine's ability to release histamine. Despite all these potential problems, codeine is an excellent and remarkably safe drug. Dextromethorphan is claimed to be as strong an antitussive as codeine, but patients don't seem to believe it and neither do I; perhaps this is because it has no sedative effect. You have to push the dose; the amount present in most cough syrups is insufficient. Figure on 3 to 4 mg/kg/24 hr divided for administration every 4 hours for infants and children, and 20 to 30 mg every 4 hours for adolescents. The long-acting preparation (Delsym) is excellent.

In medical journal advertisements, endless attention is devoted to the subject of expectorants. Apparently, the old theory of evil humors in the body is still extant, and we are supposed to want to help people to cough up sputum. This would certainly be a big help in cystic fibrosis and other chronic obstructive lung diseases, but as far as ordinary respiratory infections are concerned, this is simple nonsense. The respiratory tract produces secretions, and in most instances it gets rid of them very nicely without our help. This is fortunate, since there is no such thing as an effective expectorant. Guaifenesin, which is an ingredient of numberless cough remedies, is close to useless. Massive doses (24 teaspoons of Robitussin syrup a day for adults!) cause a trivial increase in sputum production; normal doses provide little or nothing except a foul taste.

Aside from tender loving care and lots of Kleenex, there is not much else to do for common colds. Some families give the children ascorbic acid in large amounts. There is actually a little published evidence that this helps some children to throw off a cold more quickly, but it is not an impressive effect. Aside from the occasional kid who gets diarrhea from the ascorbic acid, it is a harmless and relatively inexpensive enterprise for the parents, and it may make them feel useful.

Pharyngitis

The questions about pharyngitis that bear discussion concern (1) when to look for group A beta-hemolytic streptococcus, (2) how to look for it, (3) what other treatable pathogens exist, and (4) how to treat whatever we find.

The child with coryza, a cough, a little malaise, a low fever, and a sore throat should be treated symptomatically, if at all. The likelihood that this syndrome is due to *Streptococcus* is remote. The combination of injected conjunctivae and a red throat suggests an adenovirus and can also be ignored. During the winter influenza season the typical syndrome of initial sore throat and headache, followed by increasing cough, impressive fever, and malaise is sufficiently convincing evidence against a streptococcal infection. We need to look for *Streptococcus* when the pharyngitis and fever are the centerpieces of the illness. In middle-aged children, the first complaints are typically malaise, headache, and abdominal pain, rather than sore throat. It can be a surprise to discover a nasty-looking, red pharynx. Oddly enough, there is often little correlation between the intensity of pain and the appearance of the pharynx at any time during the illness. Tender, swollen anterior cervical lymph glands are a frequent finding with streptococcal infection. If the posterior cervical chain is swollen, one thinks first of mononucleosis.

Having decided to look for *Streptococcus,* should we use a strep antigen test or do a throat culture? The strep antigen test is one of those great ideas that doesn't necessarily work very well. False-negative results are a continuing problem with all of these products; false-positive results also can occur with some of the available brands. The promise of an instant result can be fulfilled only if a trained person is always available to stop everything else and do the test. There is also the interesting question of the wisdom of instant treatment of streptococcal infections. Some studies have suggested that the prompt use of antibiotics may blunt or obliterate the development of protective antibodies; perhaps the day waiting for the culture result is well spent. Despite all these caveats, the availability of the test is convenient for those few situations in which you would like to start treatment with more than usual alacrity. Use two throat swabs, and save one for a culture if the strep antigen test is negative. The throat culture has to be done well to be reliable. Both tonsils or tonsillar fossae plus the posterior pharyngeal wall have to be thoroughly sampled, not just lightly touched. This is no small task when a combative child is being held ineptly by a reluctant parent. It seems that a larger percentage of positive results will be found if one uses a decreased oxygen environment for incubation of the culture plates. In our office lab we experimented with a variety of techniques, including parallel cultures in room air and in increased CO_2. Our eventual compromise is to inoculate a standard blood agar plate on which we place a coverslip to decrease O_2; on either side of the coverslip we place a bacitracin disk and a trimethoprim-sulfamethoxazole disk. Many beta streptococci will show enhanced growth under the coverslip; at least 95% will be inhibited by the bacitracin, but few, if any, will be inhibited by the trimethoprim-sulfamethoxazole. The combination of findings usually allows a simple visual determination; some staphylococci will need to be differentiated either by microscopic examination or by chemical tests for peroxidase. Since we have our own lab, the results are available overnight; a negative culture can be left for another 24 hours but will only very rarely become positive.

Other bacterial and potentially treatable pathogens do occur. Non–group A streptococci certainly can cause sore throats and are easily treated with the same drugs used against group A organisms. *Corynebacterium haemolyticum* can cause pharyngitis, especially in older children and adolescents. The syndrome often includes a rash that spares the face, palms, and soles, and a cough. Discovering this organism on a standard culture may take a higher degree of bacteriologic skill than most of us have, but omitting treatment is no great tragedy. Very heavy growths of pneumococci suggest an associated sinusitis. *Haemophilus influenzae* will be found only if you use an additional culture plate of chocolate agar. If you find *H. influenzae*, what then? Is it a normal inhabitant or a pathogen? It has never made sense to me that this bacterium can cause disease north and south of the pharynx but not in the pharynx itself. However, I don't usually want to be faced with the dilemma of deciding what to do about it, so I generally don't culture for it. *Chlamydia* and *Mycoplasma* are claimed by some to cause a substantial number of sore throats. They seem to me to be in the same category as *H. influenzae*, that is, they will probably resolve without any help from me, so I don't worry about them.

Once a beta streptococcus is found it should be treated, not only to shorten the illness by a day or two but to decrease the incidence of complications. Our therapeutic choices include benzathine penicillin G given intramuscularly, which is definitive but really hurts; the mixture of benzathine and procaine penicillin G (Bicillin C-R\900–300) works equally well and is a lot more comfortable. This is a good choice if you know that a course of 10 days of oral medicine is not feasible. Oral penicillin V is fine for children who can swallow a tablet; the liquid forms taste so bad that 10 days t.i.d. becomes a real fight. In theory one can give it b.i.d., but a single forgotten dose then means a long time without penicillinemia, and the risk of treatment failure increases. Amoxicillin is a more palatable and equally effective alternative. The oral cephalosporins and clindamycin also work well, but they are decidedly more expensive. Erythromycin would be a good alternative if it did not cause so much abdominal pain and nausea; it is the best drug for *C. haemolyticum* infections.

In recent years, *Streptococcus* recurrences have become a more common problem. Most are simply due to failure to take a full course of antibiotic; finding out if the medicine was actually consumed is a good trick. I usually ask innocently, "Was there any difficulty getting him to take the entire 10 days of antibiotic?" A few recurrences are reinfections from a friend or family member; we sometimes culture the boyfriend and everyone at home searching for a carrier, but we rarely find one. The theory that *Streptococcus* may sometimes be protected by beta-lactamase–producing anaerobes or *Staphylococcus* makes sense to me. A 2-week course of clindamycin or amoxicillin-clavulanate is reasonable and usually effective. Another alternative is prolonged suppression with a single daily dose of penicillin V; several months may be required. Finally, if all else fails, consider tonsillectomy and adenoidectomy; it works.

Peritonsillar Abscess

May I be permitted a double heterodoxy? (1) All peritonsillar abscess cases do not require hospital care. If the child is not terribly ill, and that is often the case, consider penicillin G, 1 million units given intramuscularly daily, and change to generous doses of oral penicillin V (plus benzathine penicillin G for insurance, if you wish) when improvement occurs. High-dose dicloxacillin, amoxicillin-clavulanate, and clindamycin are other possibilities, especially if improvement is slow. This outpatient management works well if the family is reliable and close follow-up is ensured. It cannot be used in cases of retropharyngeal abscess, where rapid and dangerous extension can occur;

those children need a hospital and an ear, nose, and throat surgeon. (2) One episode of peritonsillar abscess does not require an interval tonsillectomy and adenoidectomy. The majority of affected kids never have another. However, if they have a second episode, I am convinced that the operation is warranted.

Otitis Externa

In 99% of cases, otitis externa is simple "swimmer's ear," the result of maceration of the skin in the ear canal by a combination of water and cerumen. The remaining cases are usually self-induced by ill-advised ear-cleaning and ear-scratching. Treatment has one crucial requirement: the canal has to be cleared of as much cerumen as possible so that the locally applied ear drops can reach the infected skin. When the patient has an exquisitely painful ear, removing the wax is no great joy for anyone. Ear, nose, and throat specialists often recommend the use of a wick to hold medication in place, but I have never found that to be necessary.

Use any of the steroid-antibiotic ear drops. The solutions tend to sting a bit more than the suspensions, but they spread more thoroughly. Special "pediatric" ear drops are not needed. Use plenty of medicine, 4 to 10 drops 3 to 4 times a day. The child should lie on one side while the drops are instilled, and he should stay in that position for at least 5 minutes, so that the medicine can thoroughly coat the canal and begin to penetrate. If he is allowed to get up immediately, the drops just run down his neck. Improvement starts in about a day. Use analgesics by mouth, if needed; otitis externa really hurts. Keep the patient out of the swimming pool until the ear is all better, usually in about a week. Avoid the products that contain acetic acid instead of an antibiotic; they are not very effective. Very rarely a treatment failure will be due to *Candida* in the canal; topical clotrimazole or similar antiyeast solutions work well.

The child who gets swimmer's ear repeatedly can be saved a great deal of discomfort by routine rinsing of the ear canals at bedtime on swimming days. Ordinary isopropyl rubbing alcohol works beautifully, probably by a combination of germicidal and drying effects. Pour a few milliliters in each ear, and let it drain right out. Another alternative is a combination of alcohol and glycerin in equal parts, but this is a little messy. The proprietary swimmer's ear prophylactic drops are also effective at 50 times the cost.

Otitis Media

One of the problems with the voluminous literature on otitis media is that careful, blinded studies of treatment require the investigators to follow rigid protocols and give up clinical judgment. Yes, I know that clinical judgment is often fallible, but that does not mean we should abandon it. I will try to make this point in the discussion of treatment options that follows. To diagnose this disorder with accuracy, one needs a clear view of the tympanic membrane. This truism needs to be stressed, because all too often we are tempted to do a little guessing or extrapolation: surely if the 50% of the typanic membrane that is visible looks o.k., we can expect the remainder to be normal as well. Unfortunately for the child, his ear canal, his parent, and our schedule, the answer is no. You have to see the whole thing. You need the brightest otoscope light available. When the battery begins to falter, the light becomes fainter and warmer in hue; everything looks a bit red. Keep in mind that some tympanic membranes light up beautifully as a result of crying; this redness is usually fairly diffuse, but the pars flaccida and the area along the handle of the malleus may look the worst, mimicking an early acute otitis media. However, the drum will move with air insufflation, without causing pain. If in doubt, leave the child to calm down for a few minutes, and then return for a quick peek. The ear should look much better if the problem was crying instead of infection. The importance of using a pneumatic otoscope is particularly great in evaluating low-grade infections and chronic ear fluid. A red-hot bulging tympanic membrane gives us all the information we need without a painful blast of air. Recently the tympanometer has been touted as a diagnostic aid; I think it is moderately useful as an adjunct to pneumatic otoscopy in the evaluation of chronic ears, but it rarely changes my treatment. It provides no diagnostic help with acute otitis media.

The diagnosis having been made, one must think bacteriologically. We can ignore the argument that viruses can cause otitis media.

Even assuming that the failure to find bacterial pathogens in every instance proves their absence, there is no way to guess which case, if any, is solely viral in etiology. There are a few clinical hints. Pneumococcus infections tend to be acute, rather than smoldering. *H. influenzae* is often the cause of combined conjunctivitis and otitis; it is more common in slowly developing otitis and especially in recurrent otitis. *Moraxella catarrhalis* is also often subacute. Beta streptococcus is a great rarity in acute otitis media, but it can cause an abruptly ruptured tympanic membrane with purulent drainage. A family outbreak of otitis can give some information; if the first child's otitis media failed to respond to amoxicillin, you would be well-advised to skip it when treating the second. It is also a help to know your current community patterns. Bacteriologic studies have shown striking differences in the flora in various parts of the world, not only in the frequency of the pathogens but in their antibiotic sensitivity. This is most striking with *H. influenzae,* which is frequently beta-lactamase–positive in some communities, so much so that amoxicillin is no longer the automatic first choice. In Spain, resistant pneumococci have been a problem for years, and this is now being seen in the United States as well. In Japan, erythromycin resistance has become common with beta streptococcus.

A less well-known phenomenon is a kind of personal idiosyncrasy of response to antibiotics. There seem to be some children for whom a given drug should work but never does. This has puzzled me the few times I have noted it; perhaps it is a problem of malabsorption. People do vary greatly in their ability to utilize drugs. In any event, when a mother tells you that Johnny doesn't seem to get any better from taking Miracle-mycin, believe her and use something else.

Which "something else" should one choose? The era of the 1960s and 1970s, when nearly every otitis could be cured with ampicillin or amoxicillin, is past. Amoxicillin-clavulanate is probably the most powerful and widely effective agent; unhappily, it does not taste good, about one fourth of its recipients get diarrhea, and it costs a great deal. Trimethoprim-sulfamethoxazole often fails against pneumococci, some brands are not palatable (Septra tastes the best but costs three times as much as the generics), and there is an increased risk of severe allergic reactions, especially erythema multiforme. Cefaclor tastes fine, but it penetrates rather poorly into the middle ear, and it is not always stable in the presence of beta-lactamases. About 1% of patients develop a serum-sickness reaction, especially if they have been exposed to cefaclor previously. Cefuroxime axetil is an excellent drug for children who can swallow a tablet easily; it is so bitter that no liquid formulation has been introduced, and a crushed tablet is ghastly. Cefixime has been promoted as a once-a-day drug, but it seems to me to be more effective when given b.i.d.; it does not work well against pneumococcus. Cefprozil and cefpodoxine are each too new to have much of a track record, and the same is true of the new beta-lactam loracarbef. Erythromycin plus sulfonamide combinations have a pretty good spectrum of activity; unfortunately the only combination on the market uses erythromycin ethyl succinate, which is not terribly well absorbed and causes a lot of bellyache and nausea. The sulfonamide is the short-acting sulfisoxazole. Better choices are erythromycin estolate (higher blood levels and less gastrointestinal trouble) plus sulfamethoxazole (longer duration of effect). Both drugs can be given b.i.d. The problem is that the patient needs two separate prescriptions, which increases cost and bother. The new macrolides azithromycin and clarithromycin may eventually prove to have advantages over their chemical cousin erythromycin.

One other therapeutic option to be mentioned is no therapy at all. This approach has two groups of advocates: a few physicians with inadequate memories of the charms of the preantibiotic era, and some anti–drug therapy parents who are similarly afflicted. Both groups may be aware of published studies purporting to show that antibiotic therapy has no effect on the course of otitis media. Among the several shortcomings of these studies are inappropriate choice of medication and inaccurate conclusions drawn by the authors.

In the enlightened community where I have practiced, a substantial group of parents seem to believe that it is a mistake to interfere with the "natural" course of a disease. Responding to this point of view in a civil and helpful manner is sometimes a strain. As a pediatrician devoted to the welfare of children, I take a certain offense at the implication that my usual mode of practice is stupid and harmful. Putting these feelings aside as best I can, I try to explain the problems of nontreatment. It is certainly true that most cases of acute otitis media subside without antibiotic treatment. We treat in order to speed healing, minimize pain, and avoid complications like chronic otitis with perforation and hearing loss, mastoiditis, and other pyogenic processes. On occasion, a parent decides against treatment and I ask that the child be brought back for follow-up every few days. If the otitis media progresses, the parent can see the necessity for treatment; one such example is usually convincing. If it isn't, I ask the family to find a doctor with whom they will be more compatible.

Having diagnosed acute otitis media, you prescribe a rationally chosen antibiotic, to be dispensed in as many containers as the child has homes or places where he will be at medicine-giving times. If he is in pain, tell the parents about the use of warmed oil in the ear. One-half teaspoon of cooking oil is heated on the stove until it is warm but not hot; it is poured into the ear canal, and a cotton pledget is placed. You can also suggest an analgesic like aspirin, acetaminophen, or codeine. Tell the family that rapid improvement is expected and that pain for more than 1 or 2 days requires a prompt reexamination.

Then what happens? In a virginal ear infection, I like to see the child in 7 to 10 days, while he is still taking the antibiotic. Most of the time, the ear looks normal or nearly so, and that is that. The child with recurrent ear infections is less likely to be cured so soon; it seems reasonable to dispense 14 days medicine and then recheck the ear. At the follow-up visit, residual ear fluid is often present. If the drum is not red, the child is asymptomatic, and there is no history of prolonged ear trouble, one option is watchful waiting; give no medicine, but look again in 2 or 3 weeks. Sometimes the fluid is gone and the patient needs nothing further. However, a pink or red ear, a purulent nasal discharge, some wet cough, continued malaise, any more earache—all these signs tell you that persistent infection is likely to be present and more antibiotic treatment is needed. In these situations, the odds are increasing that a beta-lactamase–producing bacterium is present, especially if your first antibiotic was amoxicillin.

There are certainly other causes of failure of treatment for otitis media: poor penetration of the antibiotic into the middle ear space with cefaclor and perhaps other drugs as well, pneumococcal resistance to trimethoprim-sulfamethoxazole, and, of course, failure to take the medicine as prescribed. One recent study indicated that there was a higher incidence of treatment failure when both a bacterial and a viral pathogen were present in middle ear fluid during the acute stage. There is also the major problem of eustachian tube malfunction, which can convert an acute otitis media into a chronic abscess with undrained pus. In any case, the second line of defense is a well-chosen new antibiotic delivered with a pep talk on the importance of using the stuff as prescribed.

It can take quite a long time to cure some of these kids. You may run through three or four antibiotics and many weeks of treatment. If the problem simmers down to a chronic, serous otitis, there are several adjunctive therapies to consider. The most dramatic one is a short course of oral prednisone; this dries up the middle ear and revitalizes eustachian tube function in some children. The problem is that you have to cover the risk of bacterial flare-ups with a potent, broad-spectrum antibiotic; failure to do so may cause dramatic worsening of the condition. Steroid nasal sprays can also be used in this fashion, especially if a stuffy allergic upper airway is a contributing factor.

A much milder measure that I like a lot better than steroids is inflation of the middle ear with a Politzer nasal syringe or a self-induced Valsalva maneuver. The Politzer bag is a big rubber bulb attached to a rubber tube with an olive-shaped nasal tip. One places the tip in either of the child's nostrils while pinching the other nostril shut. Then the child is told to say "kitty-kat," "cookie-cutter," or just "kay." As the sound is made, the soft palate closes off the upper nasopharynx; the Politzer bag is squeezed, and air is forced up the eustachian tubes into the middle ears. Be gentle! This hurts if done with excessive vigor. If the ears are not felt (or heard) to pop, try again. An alternative method is to have the child hold a small amount of water in her mouth and then to swallow as you squeeze the Politzer bag. This takes some practice but works well. Once a child has learned how inflation of the ears feels, she can often learn to do it herself with a Valsalva maneuver. For very stubborn serous otitis, home use of the Politzer bag b.i.d. or self-inflation with the Valsalva can be curative. You may have noted that I have omitted mention of oral deconges-tants; after using them for decades, I finally conclude that they add nothing except expense and bother.

Long-term, low-dose antibiotic use is well-established both to control frequent episodes of acute otitis and to help chronic serous otitis to subside. Extended, daily use, at least during the upper respira-tory infection season works better than episodic administration at the time of a new illness. We have used a variety of sulfonamides, including trimethoprim-sulfamethoxazole, sulfisoxazole, and sulfamethoxazole (expensive but longer-acting), amoxicillin, amoxicillin-clavulanate, and various cephalosporins. The choice of drug should be based on the child's history. There is little point to giving amoxicillin prophylaxis to a child who never gets better with amoxicillin. The use of trimethoprim-sulfamethoxazole for prophylaxis has been common for years, despite the manufacturer's statement on the package insert (and in the *Physician's Desk Reference*) that it is not indicated for that purpose. This reflects the disinclination of the drug companies to pay for the studies needed to get official Food and Drug Administration approval for an additional indication. One should certainly keep in mind that allergic reactions can occur with any sulfa drug and are probably more common with trimethoprim-sulfamethoxazole. Whatever drug is chosen, one usually gives one third to one half of the standard therapeutic daily dose; it is administered once or twice daily. In a few cases, reasonable control is obtained only with full therapeutic doses.

The use of pneumococcal vaccine against recurrent otitis has not been a great success. Some studies have suggested that the combination of pneumococcal vaccine plus prophylactic antibiotics is more effective than antibiotics alone; it is certainly worth a try.

Ear ventilation or tympanostomy tubes have had a considerable, although diminishing, vogue in the management of repeated acute otitis and chronic serous otitis. The tubes seem to decrease the number of episodes of acute otitis media in a season, and they certainly give a rapid improvement in hearing in the children whose "glue ears" cannot be cleared with medical therapy. Unfortunately, the tubes fall out, plug up, and often leave scarred, weak tympanic membranes when they are gone. As I look at the older adolescents who have had multiple ear tube placements, I often see hypermobile, floppy, irregular tympanic membranes on which I would hate to offer a warranty of long-term function. My own conclusion is that repeated acute otitis media should be handled with the thoughtful but generous use of antibiotics; chronic serous otitis media should be treated with long-term antibiotics plus the adjunctive measures noted above; ear tubes should be reserved for the rare child who does not improve with medical therapy, in particular the glue ear full of thick fluid that does not budge. Using these criteria, I refer about one child per year for tube placement. Careful follow-up, including office audiometry over many years, indicates that this approach is successful in salvaging hearing and minimizes the hazards of ear tube use.

Sinusitis

The paranasal sinuses are similar to the middle ear in the infections to which they are prone: they have the same germs, similar complications, and the same tendency to chronicity. Unfortunately, sinusitis is much harder to diagnose with precision; the sinuses have nothing analogous to the tympanic membrane. Of course, the typical picture of a full-blown acute sinusitis poses no diagnostic problem: fever; face pain; sometimes a tender, pink, puffy area below the eyes; red nasal mucosa; purulent nasal discharge or postnasal drainage; tender and swollen anterior or posterolateral cervical nodes, and leukocytosis. The milder cases are another matter. Is it an allergy, a slowly healing viral upper respiratory infection, or a low-grade bacterial sinusitis? A nasal smear for eosinophils may tell you about an allergy, but there is no other simple lab test that helps. One would expect a carefully taken nasopharyngeal culture to be useful, but they rarely differentiate a bad cold from a true sinusitis; in either case you usually retrieve a mixed flora of no diagnostic importance. Sinus x-ray films have a deservedly bad name; at a considerable cost in money and radiation, an equivocal reading is common. Computed tomographic scans provide some additional data but are hardly one's first thought for a number of obvious reasons. Ultrasonography is being used but so far without much success. One old-fashioned technique that is occasionally helpful is transillumination. By using a small but very bright light (Welch Allyn transilluminator tip) in a very dark room, one can sometimes discern differences between the paired sinuses that suggest the presence of fluid. The problems are several: one must take several minutes to dark-adapt one's eyes before anything is visible; the only standard is the contralateral sinus, so one has to judge solely on the basis of difference; and there is no way to differentiate thick mucosa from purulent fluid, because both will cut down transillumination. There is, in short, no satisfactory answer. I think we should be prepared to use a therapeutic test of antibiotic treatment as one additional method of diagnosis.

Because the bacteria are the same, treatment choices are identical to otitis. The main difference is that more prolonged therapy seems needed; 2 to 3 weeks is usual. The lack of a satisfying diagnostic endpoint remains a problem, but early relapse will signal inadequate treatment.

Laryngitis and Croup

Inflammation and infection of the larynx pose a host of diagnostic problems for the clinician. The final common symptoms of hoarseness and croupy cough can be misleadingly similar, despite quite different etiologies. An acute attack of croup with a barking cough, inspiratory stridor, and hoarseness may be nothing more than the frightening but harmless "spasmodic croup" of early childhood. These children may have started with a mild upper respiratory infection the preceding day; they awaken in the night coughing, frightened, and dyspneic. The time-honored treatment is steam. The child is held on the parent's lap in the bathroom with the hot shower running and the door and window of the bathroom closed. In 10 or 15 minutes, calm is at least partially restored and the child can be returned to bed. It is also worth giving a dose of decongestant and cough suppressant medicine. If a vaporizer is available to steam the bedroom, further episodes that night may be averted. The next day the child is hoarse but not particularly stridorous, but the following 1 or 2 nights may contain more episodes of croup.

Children who get spasmodic croup once often get it again, and families learn to handle it, but it remains a frightening event each time. Besides steam in the bedroom, a combination of codeine and an oral decongestant at bedtime seems helpful in blunting the attacks. Viral croup is similar but more severe. There is often an accompanying fever, and simple home remedies may be less useful. These are the kids whose parents call you back half an hour after the first phone call and tell you that the child has not really improved. You tell yourself that it probably isn't epiglottitis, but you know you have to have a look. On examination, the child is usually agitated and crying.

He does not sit in the neck-extended, mouth-open, and drooling posture that strongly suggests epiglottitis. Should you try to visualize his pharynx? We are all aware of the risk of a sudden complete obstruction if a patient with a swollen epiglottis is made to gag, and many of us have been taught never to look. I think this leads to un-needed x-ray films in viral croup and dangerous delays in early epiglottitis. This is the time to do a very gentle examination, using a head mirror, if at all possible, and keeping your tongue blade anterior in the mouth.

Subacute or chronic hoarseness may be due to a low-grade bacterial infection; sometimes there is an associated sinusitis or laryngotracheitis. Persistent symptoms suggest vocal cord nodules, a condition requiring ear, nose, and throat consultation.

CHAPTER 25

Chest Diseases

The management of chest infections is hampered by our inability to make clear and convincing distinctions among the various causative microbes. How do we know whether we are dealing with a virus or a bacterium, or both? The white blood count is minimally helpful. Leukocytosis with young forms hints at a bacterial cause but proves nothing. Bacterial cultures are rarely possible, because most children will not provide a sputum specimen. Lung puncture or bronchial lavage are hardly feasible as routine procedures. Bacterial antigen test results are often negative, even in the presence of actual bacterial disease. Among viral agents, one can test for respiratory syncytial virus, but timely evidence of other agents is hard to obtain. Chest x-ray films may tell us where the infection is located, but they rarely suggest the cause. In this diagnostically murky situation, we make our decisions and live with our uncertainty, a reality we may not much like but eventually learn to accept.

Bronchitis

Acute bacterial infections of the bronchi generally develop as extensions of neighboring disease. The typical story is of an upper respiratory infection or a laryngotracheitis that "settles in the chest." These children are not usually very ill, but their mild malaise; and coughing can last a long time. Examination reveals rhonchi that may clear at least partially with coughing. I don't know any useful way to differentiate these infections from the low-grade, persistent coughing and wheezing that can follow a variety of viral upper respiratory infections. This latter syndrome is probably more an irritable airway disease than a continuing infection. Furthermore, it is not easy to be sure that *Mycoplasma* is not the culprit. The tendency of *Mycoplasma* infections to occur in distinct outbreaks is sometimes suggestive.

Antibiotic choice is difficult to make. During the first few years, it seems probable that any of the ordinary bacterial respiratory pathogens may be involved. A broad-spectrum agent, such as amoxicillin-clavulanate or cefaclor, is likely to be useful. In the older child or adolescent in whom *Mycoplasma* disease is common, a tetracycline (for girls over age 7 years and boys over age 8) or erythromycin provides fairly good coverage. The new macrolide agents azithromycin and clarithromycin may prove to be even better.

Pneumonia

The causes of pneumonia are numerous, but they tend to vary with the patient's age. In the newborn period we see group B streptococcus and, less often, *Listeria,* various gram-negative rods, and *Staphylococcus.* During the next few months the syndrome of chlamydial pneumonia is common. Pneumococcus is the usual cause of severe pneumonia after the newborn period. *Mycoplasma* infections can occur at any age and become the likeliest cause of mild to moderate pneumonias after the first few years of life. Other bacterial causes like *H. influenzae,* beta streptococcus, and *Staphylococcus* are possible at any age. Of course, in immunocompromised individuals the range of potential pathogens is vastly expanded. The role of viral agents in pneumonia is varied. Influenza is a good example of how a virus may be the sole agent of a pneumonitis or may prepare the way for a secondary bacterial pathogen.

The clinical picture provides some additional information. Pneumococcal disease is not only severe, but it tends to be acute. Affected patients get sick in a hurry, and they feel and look terrible. One often finds flaring of the alae nasa, splinting of the chest, and a variety of auscultatory changes. A high white blood count with young forms is typical; not many other infections give counts well over 20,000. *Mycoplasma* pneumonia is usually but not always the opposite: slow onset, mild symptoms, not much malaise, low fever, and equivocal or negative physical findings. The white blood count is unhelpful. The chest film, if you obtain one, can look much worse than the patient.

It hardly needs to be said that pneumonias can be dangerous diseases. A severe infection may need to be treated initially in the hospital with parenteral antibiotics, fluids, and oxygen. A recent fad to be avoided is the use of vigorous physical therapy in the acutely ill patient. These children feel bad enough already without having someone pound on their chests. Happily, the vast majority of kids with pneumonia can be treated at home. Antibiotic choices are many. If the clinical picture suggests pneumococcal disease, then penicillin, amoxicillin, or a cephalosporin (except cefixime) can be used. If the child is vomiting, a first dose of penicillin G, ampicillin, or ceftriaxone can be given intramuscularly. If *Mycoplasma* is likely, use a tetracycline (for girls over age 7 years and boys over age 8) or erythromycin; azithromycin or clarithromycin may prove to be equally effective. Recovery from pneumonia is sometimes prolonged; the fever often drops slowly over a few days; malaise and cough may last 2 weeks or more. Most children should stay home from school and away from sports until they have fully recovered.

Bronchiolitis

The diagnostic problem with bronchiolitis is its differentiation from asthma. If the illness is observed from the onset, one may see the characteristic pattern of upper respiratory infection followed by fever, cough, wheezing, tachypnea, and dyspnea. The recovery of respiratory syncytial virus clinches the diagnosis. But what if one sees the child for the first time late in the illness, when the fever may have subsided, and a clear history is not obtainable? How do we decide that this is bronchiolitis rather than a first episode of asthma? If respiratory syncytial virus is absent from nasopharyngeal washings, we do not know if it was present at the beginning of the illness, whether some other viral agent is the culprit, or whether the whole illness is allergic rather than infective. The necessary conclusion is that each such illness must be managed with both possibilities in mind.

The mild cases can be managed at home if adequate parental care is available. The older child who is breathing fast and hard but can still eat and sleep is likely to improve over a week or so without any help. Aerosol bronchodilators can be tried, although home administration by unskilled parents is difficult to accomplish. Oral bronchodilators have little to offer.

Follow-up of these children can also be puzzling, since so many children develop irritable airway problems after having true viral bronchiolitis. Adequate management requires that we discover which of these wheezy kids has allergic asthma.

Asthma

Much of the confusion and disagreement about the etiology of asthma stems from the attempt to find a unitary cause for what has turned out to be a wastebasket disease. The bronchial tree has a limited repertoire of responses to irritation, whether the cause is infective, allergic, or psychogenic. Unfortunately for simplicity, the same child can wheeze from multiple causes; allergic kids can get post–respiratory syncytial virus irritable airways as easily as can kids who are nonallergic. What follows from this situation is the necessity to look for the preventable allergic factors in every child who has recurrent asthma. Are there signs of other atopic illnesses, respiratory or otherwise? A nasal smear for eosinophils, serum IgE, skin scratch tests, or a radioallergosorbent test will pick up the allergic group and point to the possibility of antiallergy management.

Some illnesses seem to generate zealotry. Diabetologists fight over the virtue of close control, and asthma specialists fight over drug treatment with a fervor that suggests religious warfare rather than scientific objectivity. Perhaps the reason in both instances is that our best efforts are none too successful. In the case of asthma therapy, the pendulum swings wildly between the various contesting groups, and the practitioner needs to take every new study and every fresh outpouring of official advice with some extra caution. The undoubted fact is that asthma morbidity and mortality have steadily increased over the last decades, during which stronger and stronger drugs have come into use.

Prior to this era, the mainstays of acute treatment were epinephrine and theophylline. Epinephrine given subcutaneously has an alpha-adrenergic effect of shrinking the bronchial mucosa and a beta-adrenergic effect of relaxing bronchial smooth muscle. Its disadvantages include stinging on injection, tachycardia, jitteriness, and vomiting. The short duration of action of regular epinephrine is avoided by the long-acting preparation Sus-Phrine. I think it still has a major place in the outpatient treatment of acute asthma. It is much easier to administer to a struggling toddler than is an aerosol, and it does not require good respiratory exchange to reach the target organ. In contrast, a substantial number of children are admitted to the hospital after a few "treatments" with nebulized drugs, which probably never got past their noses.

Theophylline is another medication that has had a bad press and is unfashionable at the moment. No doubt, it has its problems. You can't use too much of it, the liquid preparations taste awful, its onset of action after oral administration is rather slow, and some kids become miserable from its central nervous system effects. Its virtues are that it does dilate bronchi, it is available in very long-acting forms, and serum levels are rather easily monitored, making it possible to avoid toxicity. There is some evidence of synergism between theophylline and beta-adrenergic agents. The major central nervous system side effects at therapeutic levels are restlessness and irritability; these can often be avoided by the concomitant use of hydroxyzine. The once-common regimen of subcutaneous epinephrine followed by oral theophylline still has a great deal to offer.

Of course, the major change in outpatient treatment of asthma during the last two decades was the increased use of beta-adrenergic, metered dose inhalers. The instant relief that these agents afford made them very attractive to the patient, and they became the main or sole drug for vast numbers of asthmatics. The first intimation of their dangers occurred about 20 years ago when a concentrated aerosol of isoproterenol caused a number of deaths. The other preparations escaped suspicion until 1990, when the first of several studies revealed excessive numbers of deaths in patients using beta-adrenergic aerosols chronically; so far, at least two drugs, fenoterol and albuterol, have been implicated. Clearly, it is time to rethink the place of the beta-adrenergic aerosols in asthma treatment.

The systemic oral use of beta agents seems to be safe. The common side effect is central nervous system stimulation, but this is easily controlled with hydroxyzine or diphenhydramine. The limiting factor is potency; the oral agents are not very effective. In the mildest cases, you may get by with oral albuterol; the combination of albuterol plus theophylline may be enough for somewhat more severe disease. Albuterol is the longest-acting of these agents but still needs every 4- to 6-hour doses; there is a sustained-action tablet that can be used for older children.

For the chronic control of asthma, we have long had cromolyn, a drug that has never quite caught on with American physicians. This may reflect its undoubted shortcomings. Cromolyn is useless for the treatment of the asthma attack. When used for the first time as a prophylactic agent, it may take weeks or even months for full effect. There is no long-acting preparation; most patients need to use it 3 or 4 times a day. Its virtues are equally clear: practically no toxicity or side effects and a considerable degree of efficacy in controlling chronic asthma.

It is perhaps worth mentioning the use of atropine and ipratropium aerosols, although they have not yet proved to have a significant role in asthma therapy. Their current importance is as a reminder of how little we know and how sure we tend to be about our limited knowledge. For years, the revealed dogma was that any atropine-like drug had to be avoided in asthma, lest it thicken bronchial secretions. Now it seems that this is not a problem after all—so much for dogma.

The newest dogma is that asthma is an inflammatory process for which steroids are the answer, and there is no doubt that they are the strongest agents we have. One difficulty in the management of acute asthma is that steroids take effect slowly; the wheezing patient still needs one of the quick-acting drugs for the first day or so of treatment. The major problems with steroids are the long-term systemic effects. Initial studies of steroid aerosols seemed to show no significant absorption and no effect on the pituitary-adrenal axis. However, more recent investigations suggest that systemic effects do occur. Now that high-dose, chronic use of inhaled steroids is being recommended, even larger systemic effects are inevitable. The occasional use of steroids for 5 to 7 days parenterally or orally seems to be prudent and effective. What concerns me are the children who end up with frequent short courses that add up to many days per year on systemic steroids. Perhaps with perfect follow-up and compliant parents, we could always avoid excessive use. What I have seen is not so perfect: parents learn that 5 days of prednisone works like magic, and their interest in less dramatic long-term interventions is hard to sustain. The doctor on call or the emergency room doctor prescribes yet another course of prednisone, and the days of steroid exposure mount up. The eventual cost in growth retardation and cataracts 10 years down the road may be high.

Clearly there are many therapeutic options in asthma; there is no single, best treatment, but the following suggestions appear to be reasonable in our current state of knowledge:

1. Always look for allergic factors. If you can find the cat or the house dust mite or the peanut butter sandwich that increases the child's asthma, much illness and unneeded drug therapy can be avoided.

2. Nonallergic irritants, such as cigarette smoke, can be a factor. The parent or the baby-sitter who smokes may respond to your pressure to cease and desist. Even wood-burning stoves make asthma worse.

3. The child who is ordinarily free of asthma but wheezes with every cold may be helped by the prompt use of decongestants and bronchodilators at the first sign of a sniffle. This is surprisingly hard for parents to do; you may need to lean on them time after time.

4. The child who needs chronic medication should probably not use aerosol beta agents on an everyday basis. Among the alternatives, cromolyn is most effective in the well-organized family that can really manage 3 or 4 treatments day in and day out. Theophylline can be given b.i.d., and compliance is therefore a little easier. Long-acting theophylline preparations are not all the same; you may need to experiment to find the best brand. Absorption varies with food intake, so the routine of administration should be as constant as possible. Most kids do best with b.i.d. preparations; the "24-hour" capsules are not reliably absorbed, and some of the granules may come right through in the stool. Start with a small dose of theophylline and increase slowly to avoid central nervous system symptoms and vomiting. It is not always necessary to check blood levels, but unexpected treatment failure or possible toxic effects are obvious indications for testing. Erythromycin and a few other drugs increase theophylline levels.

5. It is not easy for small children to use metered dose inhalers;

the use of holding chambers is absolutely necessary. Older children can learn to use metered dose inhaler devices without a holding chamber, but this is not an easy skill to acquire and is probably not maximally effective. Someone must instruct parent and child in the theory and practice of metered dose inhaler use, and a follow-up demonstration at a later date is mandatory to make sure an effective technique is being employed. The drug companies are happy to provide placebo inhalers for demonstration and practice.

6. A special problem with nebulizer machines is the deposition of medication as droplets on the inside of the equipment. If you use a smaller volume for a small child, the proportion of medication lost will be greater. Therefore, dilute the medicine in the same volume of saline that you would use for a larger child. Because small children so often resist nebulizer treatments, you may need to use a bigger dose than you would have expected on the basis of size.

7. The treatment of asthma typically becomes complex and confusing, with different drugs being used for prophylaxis and for the treatment of the acute attack. It gets worse when multiple doctors are involved, each of whom prescribes a different regimen. It may help to give the family a flow sheet showing which drugs are to be used for what indication. An occasional spring cleaning of the medicine cabinet is not a bad idea.

8. Everyone agrees that viral upper respiratory infections trigger asthma, but there is debate about the role of bacterial infection. Perhaps we should keep an open mind about this question and be willing to use antibiotics if bacterial disease seems to be involved. Parenthetically, fever with asthma does not always mean that infection is present; one often sees a moderate elevation of temperature at the height of an asthma attack, and the fever subsides promptly as the asthma clears, with or without the use of antibiotics.

9. The miniature Wright peak flow meter is interesting and sometimes useful in the office for monitoring the course of asthma. Among the several factors that limit its reliability are variation in results, depending on which instrument one has used; we have two each of two different devices in our office, and they rarely agree. Furthermore, it is difficult to get some children to make an optimal expiratory effort. Some writers have been promoting its use by parents

at home as an early-warning system to trigger the use of asthma medication or as a guide to the severity of symptoms during an attack. I suppose there may be some families sufficiently well-organized and compulsive to master the device and to keep accurate records of each trial, but so far I'm unimpressed. Generally, both parents and physicians will do better to watch the patient, rather than the machine.

CHAPTER 26

Diabetes Mellitus

During the bad old days before insulin was available, the treatment of the diabetic child was a fatal study in medical frustration. The best advice the doctor could give the patient was to starve slowly to death on a low-carbohydrate diet. Perhaps that awful impotence was part of the reason that diabetes treatment took on the moralistic tone that still taints our current teaching. Looking at a preinsulin-era manual for diabetic children was instructive for me. It was called a *Catechism for Diabetic Children,* and it included illustrated lessons that drove home the message that diabetes had to be met by sheer willpower. In one memorable picture, a 2-year-old is proffered an apple, but the good diabetic child refuses the bad food.

After insulin was introduced, a certain degree of that Puritanism was retained. Close chemical control of diabetes was preached with a nearly religious fervor. Strict dietary rules were promulgated that required immense changes in a patient's life. Blood and urine sugar levels were commonly described as "good" or "bad"; patients were said to "cheat" on their prescribed diets. This injection into medical practice of standards and values suggestive of a theological rather than a clinical approach still persists, and it has profound and damaging effects. When we make impossible demands and then show disapproval rather than compassion, we build a wall between ourselves and our patients. They respond with anger, avoidance, and lies. One sees this most clearly in the adolescent with diabetes who forgets his urine or blood tests, fakes the results, binges on "forbidden" foods, and ends up in the hospital with ketoacidosis.

This destructive pattern can be avoided. First, set reasonable and reachable goals for the diet. We can teach the necessity of a fairly even caloric intake from day to day, the importance of avoiding massive binges of any kind, the need to cover extra calories when they are consumed, and the difficulty in handling large amounts of simple sugars rapidly consumed as snacks. Over time, a considerable degree of dietary sophistication is developed by parents and children. This should be used to increase their freedom in choosing foods. For the rare family that can follow strict dietary patterns and the rare child for whom this is reasonably comfortable, close chemical control of diabetes can be sought, even though current evidence has not demonstrated long-term gains. For the vast majority of parents and patients, the best we can hope for is enough normalization of metabolism to allow normal growth and to avoid ketoacidosis.

How often is it possible for a satisfactory dietary pattern to be fashioned within the framework of an ordinary family diet? Clearly, it is a desirable goal, because it avoids stigmatizing the diabetic child as different and sick, and it makes family eating a normal rather than a therapeutic undertaking. Unfortunately, the pattern of food preparation and consumption in many families is both unhealthy and chaotic. We all know the television image of the well-organized, middle-class, two-parent household, in which everyone eats together three times a day. What we must keep in mind is that most American families' eating patterns are basically catch as catch can. Especially in working-class households, family meals are a rarity. The reality of the diabetic child's home life must guide our dietary advice. Here is the place for a skilled pediatric nutritionist who can survey the way the family buys and prepares food and can chart an appropriate diet within those patterns.

Perhaps nowhere else in pediatric practice is the issue "Who is in charge?" more important. When diabetes appears in childhood, medical responsibility for the child's life is thrust on the parents in an extraordinarily dramatic fashion. They must learn how to test urine or blood for sugar and ketones, how to measure and administer the life-saving insulin, how to decide how much insulin to give, and how to estimate the effects of illness and activity on insulin requirements. The process of feeding the child, always heavily laden with emotional meaning for parents, becomes a medical undertaking, burdened by the thought of possible long-term effects on the child's future health.

Small wonder that the burgeoning independence of the adolescent poses particular problems for the diabetic's parents. Somehow, the parent must transfer all these tasks to the growing child and teenager. The patient must learn these skills and increasingly be trusted to make these decisions alone. The clinician can help the process by including the child, as soon as possible, in the treatment of her diabetes. Certainly by middle childhood, the diabetic should be involved in management discussions. By middle adolescence, as often as is possible the patient should see her doctor without a parent being present. This takes some doing; you may find it useful to schedule some brief talk visits for the parents, specifically to discuss these issues. For all of us parents, the prospect of our children entering the world of adult decision-making is anxiety-provoking. When those decisions are so clearly linked to life and death, it is no surprise that the parent of a diabetic child may have extraordinary difficulty with the transfer of authority.

The change is emotionally charged for the adolescent as well. As a child, she has felt the constraints imposed on her by her parents in the name of protecting her health. Her parents' concern and worry have been noted, and she may have internalized a great deal of their anxiety. Her inner struggle to reach independence as an adult has been affected by the years of unusual dependency that every child with a chronic medical problem experiences. For these young people, the leap to adult life is a particularly long one.

🍃 CHAPTER 27

Headache and
Other Tension Syndromes

It is 4:30 on a busy Monday afternoon in spring, the respiratory illness season is in full swing, the waiting room is full, and you are only 25 minutes behind schedule. Your next patient is a 7-year-old girl who sits quietly while her mother tells you that her daughter has been having pain in her abdomen for the last few months. Your heart sinks. You know that the little group in your examination room is about to embark on a long and probably frustrating journey to a fog-shrouded destination. How about the 12-year-old who cannot catch his breath? On close questioning, he turns out to be hyperventilating. What about the 15-year-old with chronic headache or the one with a dull, recurrent but alarming pain in the chest? In each of these instances you know, in your heart of hearts, that the odds are about 100 to 1 that the underlying problem is emotional. We all suffer from the same medical neurosis, the knee-jerk reaction that we must "rule out organic disease." It is a response based partly on reality; haven't we all heard that George Gershwin's psychiatrist failed to suspect his brain tumor? It has other causes as well, including a disinclination to delve into the complexities of emotional problems. In a brisk pediatric practice, who has the time to find out why this kid has a bellyache, let alone the psychiatric skills to undertake the search?

The usual way we handle these complaints is to look first for the common organic illnesses with similar symptoms. This is absolutely sensible; there are many worse approaches, including jumping to the conclusion that organic disease is absent. If our initial investigation is founded on a careful history and a thorough physical exam, we may be able to allay the family's worry and then schedule one or two brief

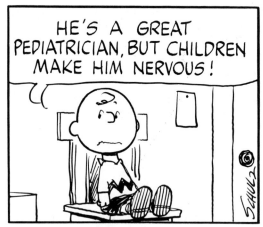

HE'S A GREAT PEDIATRICIAN, BUT CHILDREN MAKE HIM NERVOUS!

Courtesy of United Features Syndicate, Inc.

talk visits to explore the possibility of emotional tensions. On the other hand, if we immediately reach for lab or radiologic assistance, I think we set the stage for interminable searches for less and less likely entities. Furthermore, we teach the family that organic illness is the likely culprit for which we must continue searching. It is easy to fall into the pattern of more and more esoteric tests and expensive specialist consultations.

What follows from this analysis is **Grossman's First Law of Obscure Symptomatology: Trust your gut.** When faced with the kind of vague and chronic complaints that typify emotionally based syndromes, do not ask yourself what rare disease could cause this child's distress. Do not assume that a smarter doctor or one of your former professors would recognize in an instant that this is a forme fruste of Tertiary Coreopsis; it isn't. **Grossman's Second Law of Obscure Symptomatology: Remember Apley's law, which states that the closer the belly pain is to the navel, the less likely it is that the problem is organic.** There are similar hints with each somatic complaint. The chest pain that is unrelated to effort or position, the rapid respiration without wheeze and with good air exchange, the diffuse headache that never goes away—all these, like Apley's middle-of-the-belly pain, are unlikely to have an organic basis. Timing is often your best indication that a symptom is related to a situation; the Monday morning illness surely points to school, and so does week-day malaise that disappears on Friday night. Chronicity in the absence of other findings is reassuring; the unchanging headache of 5 years' duration is unlikely to have been caused by a brain tumor.

Oddly enough, the parent will probably not welcome your diagnostic impression that the symptoms are emotional. "You mean that nothing is wrong with her? I was really hoping that you would find something." This does not mean that this mom is a heartless fiend; she would simply prefer a nameable and treatable illness to the blank check of "It sounds to me as if emotional factors are behind your child's complaints." She does not want to go home and tell her husband, "The doctor says it's all in her head."

Headache is probably the most common of the tension syndromes in pediatric practice. The complaint is rare in early childhood, perhaps because little kids are not adept at localizing pain; but by school age, headaches are a dime a dozen. Some head pain is clearly a part of systemic illness, especially when accompanied by fever; this poses little if any diagnostic difficulty. Head pain can originate in several sites. Intracranial processes are the most worrisome but fortunately among the easiest to evaluate. A well-taken history, a complete physical including a screening neurologic and careful fundoscopic exams are time-consuming but sufficient. Chronic sinus infection is a rare cause of head pain in childhood. The presence of nasal congestion and discharge, tenderness over frontal or maxillary sinuses, and pain increased when the child bends his head down all point to this problem. Tooth pain or temporomandibular joint pain related to problems of tooth position are said to be a source of headache among adults. The only temporomandibular joint problems I've seen seemed to be tension-related and caused by teeth-clenching. Parents often expect headache to be due to eye problems. "Does he need glasses?" is a common question, the answer to which is nearly always "No." However, you will not be able to prove this yourself. Pediatric office testing can discover near- or farsightedness, neither of which is at all likely to cause head pain; unfortunately, we cannot diagnose astigmatism, which very rarely does seem to cause headache. I think an optometric or ophthalmologic exam is often necessary to exclude this possibility. You will soon discover that certain optometrists always find a problem, either an obscure muscle imbalance requiring expensive visual training in the optometrist's office or a minimal refractive error requiring expensive eyeglasses. One learns to pick consultants with care.

Abdominal pain of emotional origin is discussed in Chapter 22, Gastrointestinal Disorders.

Chronic fatigue and malaise form a common set of complaints in adolescence. The major symptom is usually just excessive sleepiness. The teenager comes home from school, sleeps until dinner time, and still needs more sleep at night than he has time for. Upon awakening in the morning, he usually reports feeling rested and well. Sometimes he also complains of mild, nonspecific malaise, but that is less common. His appetite is normal, and his mood may be quite good. Depending on the degree of medical sophistication of his family, he will come to you expecting the diagnosis of hypothyroidism (the favorite diagnosis of the 1960s), mononucleosis (ditto for the 1970s and 1980s), or chronic fatigue syndrome (the current favorite), none of which is at all likely. After you have performed a complete physical exam and found nothing, what should you do? Lab tests may help somewhat. Occasionally there are kids with mild hypothyroidism, so T_4 and thyroid-stimulating hormone tests are sensible. A complete blood count will pick up the iron-deficiency anemias that are common in girls. A urinalysis will tell you if there is a low-grade urinary tract infection. The remaining kids are usually in two categories: a small group with depression expressed as fatigue and a much larger group of perfectly normal adolescents. Depression usually becomes evident with further study. If you give the adolescent time to talk about his life, both he and you may find it increasingly obvious that the real problem is in his life situation. At times I find it somewhat difficult to accept this diagnosis. I tend to accept my patients' own evaluations at first, and when they present a happy face and tell me that they have not a care in the world, I want that to be true. Both doctor and patient can enter into an unspoken agreement to deny unpleasant reality. The larger, nondepressed group, truly healthy and emotionally stable, will complain of excessive tiredness for a period of weeks to months and then recover. I don't know what this means. There does not appear to be a similar syndrome among younger children, nor have I heard of this among adults. It truly seems as if certain periods of adolescent growth drain the person of energy and temporarily leave him needing unexpected hours of rest. It does not sound scientific, but there it is. A word about chronic fatigue syndrome, the newest in-vogue illness. It does seem to exist and probably has existed for a long time, having been described in the 1950s as epidemic neuromyasthenia. Differentiating it from garden-variety depression is no easy task; there is no specific clinical or lab marker for either condition, and patients with chronic fatigue syndrome are typically depressed by the illness anyway. The accompanying somatic complaints differentiate it from the benign fatigue syndrome described in the foregoing discussion.

The next problems are tactical. In the best of all possible practices, the clinician could use the first visit to enquire into the current emotional climate of the family, the parent's sense of the situation at the child's school, and the state of the child's friendships. It is hardly likely that one will have the time immediately available for that investigation; nor will the parent always be ready to share her views on such short notice. It may take a little time and reflection for some willingness to develop; you may be asking for more honesty than she bargained for when the appointment was made. You may find that the same is true when you are dealing directly with an adolescent; it can take some time for a patient to decide to look at his emotional state. Unhappily, if you do not press forward immediately, the parent or the teenager may decide to let the whole issue rest and choose not to return for further exploration. There is no easy solution to this dilemma.

In addition to bringing the parents back for talk visits, one can often talk directly with the child. Children as young as first-graders will understand when you tell them how our feelings can influence our bodies. They may be unaware of the particular emotional struggle being expressed by the bellyache or the head pain, but you can give them permission to talk about their problems and sometimes show them ways to express their feelings more directly. When the issue is anxiety related to a specific situation, one can sometimes use an awful sounding but actually playful psychological game called "Catastrophic Expectations." Either a parent or the physician can lead the patient through a sequence of imagined horrors of maximum magnitude. The child is afraid of failing a test. You ask him to imagine the very worst thing that could happen if he fails. "I'd be thrown out of school!" You ask him, if he were thrown out, what is the worst thing that could happen. "My Mom and Dad would be mad at me." You ask what would happen next. "They would make me leave home."

You continue to ask, "What next?" until the child eventually finishes the story of his downfall with, for example, death under a railroad bridge. This weird-sounding exercise has a kind of desensitizing effect: it gives an inevitably humorous perspective to the child's fears, as he is allowed to see the unlikelihood of the worst-case scenarios. Parents can use this game as often as is necessary to help a child deal with anxiety.

Older children will often understand the concept of a somatic symptom as a "message from the body," that is, a way that their bodies bring a conflict into consciousness. A verbally adept child can be asked to express the feelings in letters to or from the uncomfortable body part. This somewhat fantastical method, which might seem bizarre to an adult, makes sense to a child or an adolescent. Drawing pictures of a pain or an illness is another device that can be used.

What can the nonpsychotherapist practitioner expect to accomplish with these efforts? The main task is clarification, trying to help the parents and the child see what the likely issues might be. It often becomes clear that there has been a major and long-standing conflict within a family, with the parents in deep disagreement about the importance of a problem or the best way to solve it. In these circumstances, bringing the issue into the open may serve as the springboard for moving parents or children or both into formal psychotherapy. Surprisingly often, the opportunity to air an issue is sufficient to resolve it. The role of the clinician is to provide a supportive and neutral ground in which complaints can be expressed and solutions explored. We should not expect ourselves to solve the emotional problems of our patients. If we take on that task in the same frame of mind in which we approach the suturing of a laceration or the treatment of pneumonia, we will have arranged for our own failure. When I begin to feel myself pushed down into my chair by the weight of a child's emotional distress, I recognize this as the sure sign that I've assumed responsibility that is not properly mine. This is an important distinction between the appropriate medical roles for these two kinds of medical problems. We really are the experts who can close the laceration or cure the pneumonia, and our intervention and advice is useful and usually heeded. However, in regard to problems of human relationships and feelings, I am reasonably sure that I don't know how to live my patients' lives for them.

❧ CHAPTER 28

Migraine

Migraine deserves and gets its own chapter, separate from headaches, because it is so much more than just another kind of pain in the head. It is surprisingly common; one Scandinavian survey showed an incidence of about 1 in 20 during childhood and adolescence. The symptoms are variable, the course unpredictable, the causes multiple, and treatment neither satisfactory nor settled.

By the time I make a diagnosis of migraine, the symptoms are usually fairly obvious: throbbing headache, often (but not always) one-sided, sometimes preceded by nausea or by a visual aura, lasting for hours, and helped by rest or sleep. When I look back at the symptoms listed in my problem-oriented records, there are frequently notes dated months or years earlier about a variety of unexplained recurrent symptoms. Abdominal pain, sometimes accompanied by nausea or vomiting, is the most common precursor of migraine. Rarely, there will have been episodes of acute vertigo, lasting minutes to hours; least often, the child will have reported transient visual distortions. In young children it is particularly hard to differentiate tension headache from migraine; it may take prolonged observation to tell them apart. The strong genetic component seen in migraine is often a useful indicator. It is worth noting that some clinicians believe that tension headache and migraine are not truly separate conditions. However, patients who have migraine seem to be quite clear that the two entities are distinct.

After diagnosis, the next step is a search for the factors that trigger an episode. The literature tends to stress causes such as "let-down" migraine, which follows a period of mental or emotional

271

strain; attacks precipitated by athletic competition; the use of birth-control pills; and chronic scholastic or professional overwork. I have been equally impressed by the importance of specific food intolerances, most often of chocolate and caffeine; often a careful history or a well-kept food dairy reveals the culprits and indicates the cure.

Treatment is complicated by migraine's variability; I hate to launch a patient on a complex treatment program until it is clear that the migraine is continuing and fairly troublesome. A substantial number of patients will have only one or two episodes and then be free from further problems. So, at first I tend to treat symptomatically and await developments.

If the episodes of migraine are infrequent, it is possible to stay with the time-honored approach of rest in a dark room plus analgesics. Ibuprofen may be a bit more effective than aspirin or acetaminophen; codeine may be needed as well. The alternative is an ergot preparation; sublingual ergotamine is the simplest one and minimizes the risk of losing the medicine by vomiting. Ergotamine can also be given by inhaler, by mouth, or with caffeine by mouth. It works best if given early in a migraine attack, and, of course, the patient never has the medicine at hand when it is needed. Another vasoconstrictor, isometheptene (a constituent of Midrin), can be used if ergot fails.

For more frequent migraine, the alternatives are drugs, a large number of which have been proposed for chronic prophylaxis, or relaxation techniques, including biofeedback and autogenic training. Propranolol seems to be the best of the drugs; big doses may impair athletic performance and cause drowsiness, so proceed slowly with increasing amounts. Other beta-blockers, calcium-channel blockers, nonsteroidal anti-inflammatory drugs, ergonovine or ergotamine, cyproheptadine, anticonvulsants, and antidepressants are all used. Combinations may be needed. Any list this long implies that nothing on it works very well, and that is the case with migraine.

Relaxation techniques are sometimes dramatically effective. One can teach the patient a technique for relaxation, in which the perceived endpoint is hand-warming. It is not at all clear why this aborts a migraine, but it often succeeds. One problem with these methods is that they require more physician time to teach and to oversee at follow-up visits; I schedule a half-hour visit to explain and demonstrate, and a few quarter-hour follow-ups every other week to see how it is progressing. Another problem is parent or child skepticism; people are much more accustomed to a written prescription for a drug than to a method of body self-regulation. The payoff for the patient is a wonderful sense of mastery. My first patient who used this technique was a 10-year-old girl with a typical migraine. I had told her parents about hand-warming exercises as an alternative to her ergonovine. One night she had a severe migraine at home, and the family discovered that they were out of the medicine. They explained how she could control the headache herself by lying quietly and imagining her hands becoming heavy and warm. As she reported later, she pictured hot chicken soup running down her arms; the headache disappeared. The next morning she triumphantly told her parents, "Now I don't need to carry my pills with me anymore: I have something better inside."

The relaxation method I use, called autogenic training or autogenic therapy, is described in immense detail in *Autogenic Therapy* by J. H. Schultz and W. Luthe, published in 1969. In my simplified version, the patient is instructed to lie supine, eyes closed, and imagine or visualize the phrase "My hands and arms are becoming warm and heavy." This is continued for 2 minutes twice a day until the patient feels that an effect is rapidly achieved. One can demonstrate the hand-warming with a simple $100 biofeedback thermistor (I ordered mine from Edmund Scientific Company in New Jersey). Actually, I rarely bother with it, since the hand-warming is usually easily mastered and obvious. Once learned, the patient is to use this exercise at the first hint of a migraine. It is necessary to practice hand-warming a few times a week to keep the skill fresh; this severely limits its usefulness, because a high level of motivation and discipline is required. Sometimes a combination of medication and autogenic training works best.

Schultze and Luthe describe elaborations of this method to treat a variety of illnesses. The only other problem I have approached with autogenic training is stress-related abdominal pain; sometimes it is dramatically helpful.

❧ CHAPTER 29

Sedation and the Control of Pain

American physicians are not a particularly callous group: in general, we care about the comfort, both physical and emotional, of our patients. Unfortunately when the patients are children, their comfort is sometimes overlooked, especially by clinicians who are not primarily concerned with a pediatric age group. I saw an example of this a few weeks ago when a 6-year-old in our hospital needed a hip aspiration for septic arthritis. Her sedation and analgesic medications were inadequate, and we learned later that she was fully awake and screaming during the procedure. The orthopedist could have waited until the child was sufficiently sedated, but he didn't. Little Anna cried most of the next week; every time a doctor or nurse entered her room she was terrified. When it was time to remove her cast, the same orthopedist wanted to proceed without any sedation for her, but a vigilant house officer intervened. Anna had the cast removed while thoroughly sedated with midazolam and chloral hydrate. The nurses and doctors who take care of children must become their advocates; if we don't think about their fear and pain, no one else will.

Sedation

Ours is a country that has had a long love affair with sedating drugs. As long ago as the 1700s, travelers from Europe commented on our immense consumption of alcohol. The popular patent medicines of the last century were heavily alcoholic and often contained laudanum, heroin, cocaine, or marijuana. Not much has changed, although a variety of new agents have been added. In adult medicine, the use of sedative or tranquilizing drugs has grown apace. What are the indications for chemical sedation in children? The medical applications of these drugs are limited but important. As the case of Anna suggests, sedation before and sometimes after medical and surgical procedures is crucial. The benzodiazepines are excellent agents, safe and effective; midazolam has the added advantage of inducing amnesia, and lorazepam has the advantage of a liquid oral form. Chloral hydrate is useful if given in high enough doses; it is fairly long-acting. The liquid preparations come in a reasonably palatable wild cherry flavor and a disgusting anise flavor, which should be avoided at all costs. Barbiturates have fallen out of favor for good reasons; children often become paradoxically excited by them. I once gave phenobarbital to a family for use with their 2-year-old on a long airplane trip. As the mother told me later, through gritted teeth, "I had to walk her all the way to South Africa." The phenothiazines are powerful but rarely indicated. Chlorpromazine (Thorazine) has been used in the "lytic cocktail" of Demerol, Phenergan, and Thorazine (DPT), but this is more toxic and less effective than combinations of hydroxyzine or diphenhydramine with either morphine or meperidine. Last but not least, alcohol is widely available and can be quite useful in a pinch.

I don't mean to imply that drugs are the sole method of preparing a child for a procedure. Explanation beforehand can make an immense difference. One uses pictures or puppets or whatever is appropriate for a given child. For major elective procedures, a guided tour of the hospital is effective preparation. None of this is likely to be either quickly or simply managed; someone has to devote time and effort to the enterprise. Hospital-based child development specialists, usually referred to as "child life specialists," are specifically trained to prepare children for medical and surgical procedures and to help them handle their feelings and fears through brief play therapy. In the case of Anna, mentioned earlier, a child life worker saw her and her mother every day and helped her emotional recovery. A nurse, doctor, or social worker might undertake the same kind of effort.

Nonmedical indications for sedatives in childhood exist but are not common. It is nearly always a mistake to use drugs as they are used in adult medicine to treat anxiety, insomnia, and the other psychological miseries of everyday existence. The implicit lesson of this kind of use is that peace or happiness comes out of a bottle and that the slings and arrows of outrageous fortune can be deflected with drugs. Another lesson for the child is the ego-weakening implication that one's parents believe that one cannot cope with a problem. The child who is upset by a death, worried about a divorce, or otherwise needing support in a life crisis should be provided with an opportunity to talk to a friend, a family member, or a practitioner, not fobbed off with a drug.

Control of Pain

Let's look first at the nondrug methods of relieving pain. The simple provision of immobilization of an injured part, ice on a sprain, or a dressing over a painful burn is welcome first aid for pain. At the psychological level, careful and complete explanations can sometimes lower anxiety so that pain can be borne more easily. Talking is no panacea, but its effect should not be underestimated. Hypnosis is, in effect, a potentiated form of talking; by using normal human suggestibility it is often possible to moderate pain to a surprising degree. This technique has been used with considerable success in the management of burns and the chronic care of cancer. In a similar vein, one can teach visualization techniques that allow a patient to feel that he has a role in the management of his own disease. I think that many of us are put off from hypnosis, visualization, and related methods by the overblown claims sometimes made in their behalf. Unfortunately, more than the usual amount of self-delusion is manifested by writers interested in these modalities. Because these authors are sometimes both antiscientific and antimedical, it can be difficult for us stodgy doctors to wade through the chaff to find the wheat.

The drug therapy of pain is easily stated as **Grossman's Tripartite Law of Pain Medication: Give the right drug; give a big enough dose; give it often enough.** What appears to get in the way of following this law is underestimation of the amount of pain the child is experiencing. Especially when the patients are very young, the nonspecific crying of sick or injured children may be somehow overlooked as a sign of real pain. One sees this most commonly with otitis media, a truly painful affliction, if you can remember your own childhood. An analgesic is rarely suggested as part of our management of this disease, but if my ear were infected, I would want something for it. Actually, I think we physicians systematically underestimate the pain caused both by disease and by our treatments. It is as if we do not want to admit that we inflict pain; nor do we want to face the reality of the pain attendant to disease. An unconscious and not very helpful part of us acts as our own mothers acted when they wanted our pain to go right away. "I'll kiss it and make it better" is a combination of tender loving care and outright denial.

The issue of giving enough analgesic medication arises most often in relation to the child with serious, chronic, or fatal disease, for whom our fear of fostering drug addiction stays our hand. Clearly, if a child is dying with a painful disease, the concern about addiction is bizarrely unrealistic; this child is not going to survive to become an addict, and her pain should be relieved. Furthermore, we need to remember that tolerance to narcotics can develop, necessitating increasing doses to obtain adequate analgesia. The risk of addiction in the treatment of acute pain in childhood is close to zero; when the burn has healed or the postoperative pain is gone, the child is done with the drug. If narcotics have been used for a substantial number of weeks, it may be necessary to decrease the dose slowly, about 10% per day, to avoid withdrawal symptoms. The situation in which addiction is a real risk is in the case of a recurrently painful condition, such as sickle cell disease. Here one watches for signs of addiction, uses non-narcotic modalities when possible, and decreases drug use as quickly as one can.

Inadequate frequency of dose is the last impediment to adequate pain relief. If pain is continuing, the analgesic drugs should be given regularly, often enough to prevent the breakthrough of pain. A p.r.n. order means that the child begins to feel pain, makes this clear to the adult caregiver, eventually gets the medicine sometime later, and has unmasked pain until the next dose takes effect. That can add up to many hours of pain every day. Given on a regular basis, the analgesic will work more effectively, usually at a lower total dose, and the child can be kept much more comfortable. It takes a smaller dose of narcotic to prevent pain from recurring than to control pain after it is present. In a busy hospital p.r.n. orders for pain are particularly ill-advised. Be realistic about the duration of action of these drugs; watch the child to see how long a given dose really works.

For mild pain, aspirin and acetaminophen remain the standards. Aspirin has become a nearly forgotten drug among young parents and young physicians worried about Reye syndrome. Keep in mind that the connection, tenuous at best, is claimed only for aspirin given in the presence of influenza and chicken pox. When those entities are absent, we can still use aspirin happily for the tasks it does so well, especially joint pain and pain associated with inflammation. Aspirin has the advantage of tasting good in a chewable or dissolvable tablet, in contrast to the much less palatable acetaminophen. Besides its nasty taste, acetaminophen has only one major disadvantage: its utility as a means to suicide. In Great Britain acetaminophen has been the most popular mild analgesic for years and is now also the drug of choice for self-destruction. Recent reports suggest that chronic, daily use is associated with renal damage in adults, but so far there is no known renal problem in children. Because acetaminophen is a close chemical relative of phenacetin, long suspected to be a kidney toxin, this bears watching. Acetaminophen has the advantages of no effect on blood clotting and very little gastrointestinal irritation; when children vomit the liquid formulations, it is because of the bitter taste.

The nonsteroidal anti-inflammatory agents have earned a major role in pain control. For many types of pain, they appear to be somewhat stronger than aspirin or acetaminophen. Certainly for dysmenorrhea and arthritic pain they are often the best choices. Unfortunately, this increase in efficacy is purchased at a cost of increased toxicity, most often gastrointestinal irritation, bleeding, and ulcers, but also a variety of central nervous system symptoms, rashes, and hematopoietic changes. Each newly introduced drug is promoted as the best thing since sliced bread, and each reliably proves to have its own set of toxicities. Ibuprofen is surely the most widely used of these agents. It is a propionic acid derivative with aspirin-like actions. Drowsiness and gastrointestinal irritation are the most common problems. Another agent of the propionic acid family is naproxen, which has a long half-life and can be given b.i.d. These two drugs are available in expensive suspension form for children who need their particular virtues, but there is simply no good reason to substitute them for aspirin or acetaminophen for ordinary indications.

Codeine is discussed in some detail in Chapter 18 in minor injuries. It is not a powerful analgesic agent, but when used in full doses along with aspirin, acetaminophen, or a nonsteroidal anti-inflammatory drug, codeine can handle most pain of moderate intensity. For practical purposes it is nearly always used orally in a combination form with another drug, thereby avoiding the necessity of triplicate prescriptions. Codeine can be used parenterally; it is about one third more effective by that route. Don't ask too much of codeine by mouth; it will dull an earache, but it will probably not suffice for a major fracture.

Hydrocodone (dihydrocodeinone [Hycodan]) is basically identical in its clinical activity to codeine, but it is about twice as potent, milligram for milligram. This confers no particular advantage to anyone except the manufacturers, who charge much more for it. It is commonly prescribed in combination with acetaminophen (Vicodin) by physicians who are unaware that codeine and acetaminophen (or codeine and aspirin) would be equally effective.

For severe pain the major narcotics are meperidine (Demerol), morphine, methadone, and opium tincture. Meperidine has been a pediatric favorite for many years; it is nearly as potent as morphine, is available in a convenient multiple-dose vial, and is familiar to us because of its common use during childbirth. The duration of analgesia is shorter than equivalent doses of morphine, perhaps 2 or 3 hours on the average; this limits its utility for the control of long-lasting pain. Oral use is about 25% to 40% as effective as parenteral use. Morphine remains the standard narcotic drug. In everyday outpatient pediatric practice one will rarely need it, but for severe and chronic pain it is the first choice. It has a duration of action of 4 hours or more. Because morphine given orally is largely destroyed by first-pass degradation in the liver, oral doses are usually six times the equivalent parenteral dose. However, the bioavailability can vary wildly, from 15% to 49%, so that an individual patient's requirement cannot really be predicted. The pragmatic rule is to administer enough to control pain. One way around the first-pass degradation problem is to give the morphine sublingually in a tablet form.

As an analgesic, methadone is much like morphine, although with long-term use there may be a somewhat longer duration of action per dose. Given orally, it is much more reliably utilized than morphine; an oral dose of methadone is about 50% as active as a parenteral dose.

The advantage of tincture of opium (laudanum) for oral use is that it is concentrated. For practical purposes it is basically a 1% morphine solution, supplying 10 mg of morphine per 1 ml. Paregoric (camphorated tincture of opium) should be mentioned only to warn against its use: it tastes absolutely foul and is exceedingly dilute, providing $\frac{1}{25}$ the potency of the tincture. It is hard to understand why this medieval mess is still manufactured.

❧ CHAPTER 30

Chronic Illness and Fatal Illness

Chronic Illness

Every kind of medical practice has its characteristic mix of acute and chronic problems. The geriatricians' daily work is heavily weighted toward chronicity, and I suppose they become used to seeing patient after patient with permanently disabling pathologic processes. At the other extreme, those of us who work with children see vast numbers of acute problems—infections, rashes, injuries, and the like. Even the psychological problems we see often present as acute crises. Perhaps the brisk pace of pediatric problems is one reason we choose this field: we can expect the majority of clinical situations to have a fairly clear-cut beginning and a foreseeable end. Most pediatric diseases do not continue forever.

Unfortunately, some diseases do continue, and even worse, some go on to a fatal conclusion. These illnesses may find us, in a certain fashion, unprepared and even unwilling to adapt our expectations and our styles of practice to the different needs of the family and the child with chronic or fatal disease. We are so accustomed to thinking of "cure" that we cannot easily think in terms of "care." My own experience is that when I have seen a patient with rheumatoid disease, a static neurologic handicap, or incurable cancer I feel defeated and impotent. The patient leaves my office without the message I always expect myself to give: "You are going to get better." Now I know that this is nonsense; the family and the child have long since given up the expectation of hearing that message. Even worse, this inappropriate frame of mind is destructive of good medical practice. It makes me less eager to see the patient again, probably less emotionally present for the child and family, and more willing to abdicate my role to a specialist somewhere else.

Of course, the whole issue of generalist-specialist relationships is a can of worms, in any case. Even when I don't have the problem of the patient with an incurable disease, there are always complexities. Whose role is whose, when do you want to keep the ongoing care in your own hands, what do you do when your consultant order a line of investigation that sounds foolish to you? These are just a few examples. Recently an allergist initiated unasked for treatment for an infection in one of our patients, got all excited about a subsequent rash, and sent the child off to a costly and unnecessary visit with a dermatologist. One hesitates to put out a contract on a colleague or even to complain to him; after all, we will use him again, and who needs hurt feelings and enemies? However, in a primary care practice it is the task of the primary physician to set the rules: this is what I need for my patient, this is how follow-up care should be arranged, and this is when I'll send the patient back for more of your help. You can do this in your initial referral letter and save everyone grief. This implies the existence of an old-fashioned, formal letter of referral. A telephone call is rarely an adequate substitute; there are too many details that may get lost. Simply telling the family to see Dr. X is asking for trouble: misunderstandings about the history of the problem and lack of clarity about your expectations of the consultant's role are inevitable. When the problem turns out to be important and long-lasting, intelligent collaboration among the physicians involved becomes crucial, sometimes a matter of life and death.

When the doctor's role is "care" rather than "cure," an increasing part of medical task is support of the family. Often this is no more complicated than making time available for the parents to talk about living with a sick child. I will never forget the quiet Sunday afternoon when I was the admitting resident and a 5-year-old girl with cystic fibrosis came in. The parents provided a detailed history, and then I asked them how they were coping with their daughter's illness. Out poured a torrent of heartfelt misery. Their lives were consumed by her illness, their savings spent on it, their energy drained dry. "We have no money for a rug on the floor, no time for the other children, we worry about her all the time. We don't even make love anymore."

The child or adolescent also needs a willing listener. It can be difficult for the patient to maintain any sense of the person underneath the mask of illness. There is a danger of being self-defined as the sickness: "I am an arthritic" rather than "I am a person who has arthritis." For the growing person who is in the process of finding or making an identity, the illness may overshadow everything else. During the years of middle childhood and later, when being like one's peers is painfully important, the demands of the illness and its intrusion into everyday existence may become intolerable. One common and dangerous reaction is to deny the illness; these are some of the kids who end up in diabetic ketoacidosis or status asthmaticus. Giving them a chance to talk about their lives and to complain to you about how hard it is to be limited by a disease can be life-saving. We can't cure the diabetes or the asthma, but we can let them know that we understand and we care. Patient support groups can also play an important role. Just being with others who are confronting the same problems is immensely useful. "I'm not the only one with this" can make coping with illness a lot easier. Of course, support can come from many other sources as well; psychotherapists, home health aides, special education teachers, and physical and occupational therapists.

Family support is likely to include the other children. From the viewpoint of his brothers and sisters, the child with a chronic disease gets far more than his share of attention from the parents and everyone else. *He* gets to stay home from school, *he* doesn't have to do his share of the chores, *he* is the one friends and relatives make a fuss over; the price he pays for the advantages of illness is not noted. The healthy sibling often wishes that his sick brother or sister were dead and feels guilty and angry about his guilt. If the patient dies, the sibling may blame himself, especially during the earlier years of magical thinking. It may be possible to forestall some of this by alerting the parents to the problem or by talking directly to the other kids about what a pain it can be to have a sick person in the family. Another common response to family illness is the "sick sibling syndrome," a set of complaints that tend to be vaguely reminiscent of the other child's real illness. These symptoms may occur at any time during the illness or as anniversary symptoms after a child's death. Don't confront this head-on; give the healthy sibling some room to develop an understanding of what is going on without feeling like an unmasked fraud.

Fatal Illness

Some patient's questions are never forgotten. An 8-year-old boy with a malignant brain tumor was nearly completely paralyzed; he could hear and he communicated by blinking his eyes in response to his parent's pointing to letters on a board. One day at the end of a visit he asked me, "Am I going to die?" It was a question for which I was wholly unprepared. I had no idea what he had been told by his neurosurgeon and his parents. How much could he understand about death? He watched me and his parents watched me while I hesitated and then responded, "Yes, you are going to die. There is no medicine that can make you better." That was about 25 years ago, and the memory still hurts. I am your doctor, and I cannot help you to live. It is partly in order to avoid that implicit question and its terrible answer that we physicians tend to stay away from the dying child. A number of years ago, a careful study measured the length of time doctors and nurses spent in the rooms of dying children; the sicker the child, the less time the doctors stayed. The nurses, whose role is defined as caring rather than curing, did not have to avoid contact with the children whom the physicians perceived as their failures. The implication is clear: if we are to help the child with a fatal disease, we must, in part, redefine our expectations of ourselves and our professional roles. We cannot always cure, but we can always help.

There are no formulas, decision trees, or algorithms to guide us in this area. Obviously, the intelligent use of drugs can reduce pain and can control many of the symptoms of illness, but many larger questions remain. How is the decision made to subject a child to last-ditch therapies with no real prospect of success? Sometimes this question can be faced when the child is at home, the parents have time to consider all the aspects of the choices being offered, and the child's own wishes can be weighed. This hardly blunts the painfulness of the decision, but it at least allows the people involved to retain some control. Unhappily, most such times of decision arise in hospitals, where there is rarely enough time for complete explanations, the pressure to do something is omnipresent, and lines of authority are blurred. Who is in charge of the child? The parents are frightened by the illness, confused by the hospital environment, and overawed by the complexity of treatment. The primary doctor has often stepped back from direct management of the case, deferring to the specialists, and the specialists may be squabbling among themselves about how to proceed. It is easy to lose sight of the patient. In this situation, the pediatrician must reclaim the role of advocate for the child and the family. If the hospital has a medical ethics committee, it may need to be asked for help as well. Otherwise, decisions may be made on the basis of which consultant has the loudest voice.

"Am I going to die?" At some point in many illnesses, we have to face that question. The paternalistic physician of an earlier era knew that the question should not be answered directly, if at all. One was supposed to keep up hope at all costs, even though that meant lying through one's teeth. For myself, the need to maintain an honest relationship with the family and the patient is so powerful a rule that lies and evasions are nearly impossible to countenance. When push comes to shove, lying means that you do not trust the patient to handle reality, and your lies make it impossible for them to do so. This can hardly be in anyone's best interests; bite the bullet, and tell the truth.

When a fatal illness is prolonged, the pressures on the parents and other children and family members become unbearable and terribly destructive. Marriages are often destroyed, family relationships often blighted. The grinding necessities of taking care of the dying child will burn out the most dedicated parents. To some degree this can be prevented by the provision of help from the outside. This may come from extended family and friends supplemented by paid household caregivers or volunteer hospice workers. Initially, parents may not be ready to accept external support, because they believe that they can and should provide all the care by themselves or because they have not yet accepted the reality that their child is dying. The physician can help with this process by explaining the necessity from the larger point of view of the needs of the whole family, and, in effect, giving the parents permission to seek and accept assistance. We can also make sure that the family knows about the social services available in the community. This may also be the time to make a referral to a psychotherapist skilled in counseling dying patients and their families.

Death has become a hospital event in recent years. Sometimes the setting is determined by the nature of the illness, and death may have to arrive in an intensive care unit or on the ward, with all the medical paraphernalia of tubes and machines and codes. This is the worst possible situation for everyone. It often leaves the family pushed to one side by last-minute heroics, with no place to go and no way to say good-bye. Hospital deaths can be a nightmare to be remembered forever. If the child can be allowed to take leave of life at home, there is at least a chance that the last hours can have some modicum of peace for the patient and his family. It takes careful arranging and is easily disturbed. If a panicked caregiver calls 911, horrifying and pointless efforts may be made to revive a moribund child. If the family has not been taught how death may come, they may be too frightened to cope with what they see. But at least in some circumstances, the death of a child in his own bed in his own room with his own family can be a healing event in the family's process of grieving.

For me, there has been nothing harder in pediatric practice than the visit with the parents a few weeks or so after the death of the child. I think we owe them this opportunity to review whatever they wish concerning the illness and to talk about how they and the rest of the family are coping. Parents need to know that the process of mourning is exceedingly long; they may expect to somehow have surmounted their grief and be back to "normal" within a short time, but that will not be the case. The experience of a child's death will change forever the way parents deal with disease. Every subsequent illness in the other children will stir anxiety all out of proportion, but this is easily understood. The focus on the survivors can become quite pathological. One of the most hazardous paths a family can take is to have a "replacement" child. It is a way to shortcut grieving for the child who died, and it means that the new child is burdened with parental fears and expectations that have nothing to do with him. Counseling against a prompt pregnancy may be the best advice the parents will ever get.

Thinking about the role of the primary physician in these situations of chronic and fatal disease makes it clear how broadly we can define ourselves as the helpers of children and families. As listeners, as guides, and as supporters in hard times, we can make an immense difference in the lives and deaths of children and families. Even when our efforts do not cure disease or prevent death, we can still be valuable and deeply appreciated doctors for children.

CHAPTER 31

Schools and Learning

Abraham Flexner was the man who revolutionized American medical education. The study of medical schools that he carried out for the Carnegie Foundation early in the twentieth century forced the profession and its academic leaders to restructure our schools on the basis of the scientific, German model. Later, at the conclusion of a brilliant career, he founded and directed the Princeton Institute for Advanced Study. In his autobiography he described his own primary school education: "Such was the schooling of that day that we were almost as free from intellectual strain, effort, or interest during school hours as during the long Southern afternoons and evenings." About high school he said, ". . . some of the teachers were incompetent, and others were unable to preserve discipline in the classroom. . . . Good teachers were scarce."

I think of Flexner every time I see the furrowed, worried brow of a mother or father who is agonizing over the importance of admission to the best nursery school. The current middle-class preoccupation with the minutiae of primary education is fascinating but depressing. It is based upon an underestimation of the contributions of the family, on the one hand, and the child, on the other. From the family the child learns whether learning is desirable, whether questions can be posed and answered, whether books are valued, and whether one must sometimes work quite hard to reach a distant goal. The child brings her own styles of thought, patterns of activity, ability to focus, interests in the world, pecularities of temperament, and most important, her own particular brain, with whatever neuronal organization it has been blessed. With these raw materials the schools and teachers must struggle.

Of course, the "right" school has been important for a very long time, but in the past this mostly meant schools with the proper upper-class cachet. Reading biographies of the people who attended the best schools reveals a pattern of nearly unrelievedly dreary, rigid, and pedestrian instruction. One met the right people and learned the styles of the well-to-do; studies were clearly secondary. The emphasis now is somewhat different; schools are chosen to get the child off on a running start in the race of life, but the academic experience itself is thought to matter mightily. But does it? A revealing study of general practitioners in North Carolina compared the quality of their medical work with the places of their medical training. It did not matter a bit where they had studied: Harvard graduates were not distinguishable from the doctors from West Nowhere State.

I don't want to push this argument too far. Certainly one wants one's child to flourish in a beautiful and happy classroom, taught by eager and bright teachers with skill, love, and compassion. Certainly one wants one's child to have adequate exposure to the full range of intellectual fare, with all the bells and whistles of computers, slide projectors that work, and a wonderful playground; but there is more to school than all that. What one learns first and foremost in primary school are (1) who is in the world and (2) how they treat one another. A friend of mine who grew up during the 1930s in Brooklyn told me that as a child, he thought nearly everyone in the world was Jewish. On the rare occasions when he met a gentile, he felt terribly sorry for him because he thought it must be so lonely. A teenaged patient of mine had recently moved to a lily-white suburb from his previous residence in our multiracial city. I asked him what the kids were like in his new high school and he replied, "The only black they ever see is the janitor! They're all afraid to come to Berkeley to go to a movie!" In short, the local environment, of which the school is so important a part, shapes and limits our world view. As parents abandon public education in order to obtain the "best" for their children, they choose a narrowing environment, one that feels comfortable and safe but insulates the child from the realities of contemporary American life.

One must use some judgment in all this; some of those realities are clearly too dangerous for any child. Nevertheless, some are not, and they provide the opportunity to cope, to test oneself against adversity and difference. We all need survival skills, and we get them only through practice; we learn to be street-smart on the street. Without that exposure we remain naive or frightened, or both.

Apart from these large and difficult social issues, there are innumerable times when a given child is not happy or thriving in a given classroom. The parent's protective impulse may be to move the child to a different class, but if the problem is intrinsically that of the child himself, a change of scene will not be the answer. One needs to ask what the child brings to the classroom. It may be his own anxiety, his lack of social aptitude, his unhappiness about a situation in his home, or the first signs of a learning disability. When I am asked for my opinion about dealing with such a problem, I need a considerable amount of information to sort this out. A telephone call to the teacher is the first step. The classroom teacher is delighted to hear from a child's doctor; if the child is having trouble, so is the teacher, who will appreciate help. The viewpoint of the teacher is always useful as a part of the diagnostic picture one is building. Parenthetically, I have learned to be wary of the diagnoses teachers proffer. They are not taught to think in diagnostic terms, and they easily mistake the symptom for the disease.

If a school psychologist is available, it is often possible to arrange either formal testing or informal classroom observation; both are useful. Watching and talking with the child in the office are obviously helpful as well, but the situation in a school classroom or on a playground is different from the quiet, one-to-one meeting in your office. Especially when the problem turns out to be hyperactivity or attention deficit disorder, it is easy to be misled. At times, the only way to gain clarity is to bring everyone together at the school. This kind of case conference can be invaluable.

Learning Disabilities

This discussion should have the subtitle "A Tragicomedy." Learning disabilities, sometimes associated with problems of attention and behavior, have been the subject of study since the early decades of this century. The depth of confusion regarding causation is matched only by the proliferation of nonsense regarding treatment. Nomenclature changes every decade, at least; "dyslexia" became "minimal brain damage," which became "minimal brain dysfunction," which became "attention deficit disorder," which became "attention deficit–hyperactivity disorder," at least part of the time. The theory of the importance of mixed laterality (that is, the dominant hand was not on the same side as the dominant eye or foot) was promulgated by researchers who did not notice that mixed dominance was equally common in kids with no learning problems. Treatments were invented that claimed to retrain the brain into more normal patterns by teaching the children to crawl "properly" or to walk on a balance beam with greater grace. At the same time, drug therapy became popular as a method to make the children more tractable, even if it didn't seem to do much for their eventual intellectual functioning. In diagnosis and therapy, a thousand flowers bloomed, but, alas, now have mostly faded.

We are left with a rather small store of what appears to be reliable information. Incidence figures are terrible. Because girls with problems of attention and learning tend to be quieter and cause less trouble than similarly afflicted boys, the girls are often overlooked and underdiagnosed. The sex ratio is not the 4 to 1 quoted in the literature; it may be nearer 1 to 1. Anatomic and physiologic studies show that indeed these kids' brains are wired differently; this should give pause to anyone with a quick-fix panacea. Ordinary medical and neurologic examinations are either wholly useless or, at most, reveal a modest excess of "soft" neurologic signs, which are often just a measure of immaturity. You can't hang your hat on them. Observation of the child in his normal habitat by teachers, parents, psychologists, or physicians may reveal short attention span, impulsivity, distractibility, irritability, physical awkwardness, or nothing at all. Psychoeducational tests are the best single tool to define the learning problem per se. This obviously requires a skillful psychologist who will not be misled and distracted by variations in behavior and functioning due to class and ethnic differences.

In short, when a child in the early years of school is doing poorly, one needs to ask whether this is because of a ghastly classroom situation; subcultural differences in expectations; a destroyed home life; a major or minor disorder of psychological health; simple mental deficiency; a specific disorder of reading, speech, or motor activity; poor vision or impaired hearing; attention deficit disorder; or any combination of the foregoing. It is a fairly long list but not too hard to winnow. Take your time, get some help from a good psychologist, don't let the family fall into the hands of the 15 varieties of quacks who prey on these kids, and don't be in any hurry to reach for your prescription pad.

You should also keep a firm grip on your expectations of cure. The children who have a specific learning disability without attendant problems of attention and behavior benefit modestly from the best special education programs. It is as if they learn alternative ways to do the mental work required. In later life they often continue to have the same basic difficulties; their reading or spelling or whatever may never amount to much. This is not always a disaster. One father whose son had dyslexia told me that he had the same problem: "All through Harvard law school my reading was so slow that I had to hire other students to read the cases aloud to me." The children with problems of behavior continue to struggle with the same impulsivity and distractibility that made their teachers and parents want to strangle them years before. As adolescents, they often still behave in a more acceptable and civilized fashion when they stay on their methylphenidate or dextroamphetamine; it is difficult to know when it should be discontinued, if ever. Their futures may contain more episodes of delinquent and criminal behavior than anyone wants to contemplate. This is not always the case, fortunately, and one should not predict an end on the gallows; the parents have enough to cope with as it is.

CHAPTER 32

Television and Other Distractions

If one spends a few moments asking parents how their kids spend the day, it becomes clear that a bombardment of electronic noise is present from infancy onward for many hours every day for the vast majority of American children. Babies are propped in front of the colorful noisy feast of TV, toddlers play with TV blaring in their ears and eyes; all kinds of programs fill the rooms where older children and adults live their lives. Some of this is background for the main activities of the day, and some is the focus of rapt attention; all of it has an effect.

One of the effects of home video games and the portion of TV that is actually watched is substitution: what would this child be doing if the TV or the Nintendo were not there? As our children get fatter and softer, it is obvious that a substantial amount of physical playtime is lost. This should come as no great surprise; children are awake about 12 to 16 hours a day, and school kids are away from home for about half of that time. The few hours of daylight that remain after school are easily invaded by the tube. Reading and school homework are also obvious candidates for eclipse. After one or two favorite programs are watched following dinner, it's nearly time to go to sleep. When does the homework get done? When does the family have focused time together without the distraction of TV? Do people still read to their kids?

One mother I know became alarmed about the invasion of Monday night football, situation comedies, and cartoons; she took the unusual step of disabling the family TV and announced to everyone that the repairman had the necessary part on back order. The results

295

were instant. Books were read, craft projects undertaken, noisy and active outside play resumed, and father and children had meaningful time together. After 2 months, the TV was "repaired," but stringent rules for viewing kept the beast at bay. It was one of the most useful lies I've ever observed.

One of the other effects of TV is a perfect example of Marshall McLuhan's dictum that the medium is the message. TV's intrinsic message is "Expect excitement and entertainment, even learning, without any effort at all." The effect of bathing in this culture of passivity is reported by primary school teachers who say that the TV-reared child is easily bored by the monochromatic, quiet effort required to master basic skills.

The explicit messages of TV's content, both programs and advertisements, is another matter. I suspect that most of us are so inured to it that we are hardly aware of the underlying ideas, which can be summarized as follows: (1) People are fools. Attractive, coherent-sounding human beings have so little sense that they get excited about the effectiveness of a floor polish, celebrate the delights of a soft drink, and act as though a hair rinse were changing their lives. (2) Consumption is what really counts; that is the royal road to happiness. (3) Sexual intercourse is generally devoid of consequences. One must be ready for sex at any time, it is mistily and deliriously passionate, and nobody ever seems to get herpes. (4) Violence is the royal road to survival. Expect life to be filled with knives, fists, guns, and a variety of other explosives. Killing people is not very important; they just fall down and die. It doesn't generally seem to matter much to anyone.

Violence is now attractively packaged for our children in home video games such as Nintendo. In case you have been hibernating for the last decade and missed this, the basic scenario is violent confrontation of enemies. It is the player's task to destroy, that is, kill, the enemies. That is what the game is about: becoming a competent killer with good eye-hand coordination. One of my partners described a new game to which a friend had introduced her children. The story line was simplicity itself; three teenaged gangs (yellow, white, and brown) fight each other on a high-school playground. They use switch-blade knives and other academic tools to kill each other. The winner is rewarded with the girlfriend of the murdered leader of the defeated gang. When my horrified partner returned the video game to the store, the clerk said dismissively, "It's certainly getting harder to be politically correct here in Berkeley."

Does any of this matter? There can hardly be any doubt about the immediate and powerful effect of TV on children. A number of studies have demonstrated that experimental exposure to TV violence is followed by an abrupt increase in violent behavior among the children. It is true, of course, that Americans have always had a violent society, addicted to guns, celebrating aggression, making heroes out of our outlaws. For the last half century or more the world has been an incredibly violent place, never for even 1 year being free from wars. Since the Vietnam War, we have brought war into our homes with the evening news. Our politics and our entertainment are in complete agreement; both systematically teach our young to expect and therefore to accept killing as the norm. They learn fast: homicide is now the second leading case of death from age 15 to 35 years.

We pediatricians realize the limits of our influence; none of us relishes the role of King Canute, lashing back the tides. However, we can help families to look critically at the immoral and destructive content of our children's entertainment and at the Gresham's law effect of harmful activities pushing out the good ones.

CLINICIAN: "How many hours is Betsy awake during an average day?"

MOM: "Well, she sleeps from 9:00 P.M. to 7:30 A.M., and she takes a 1-hour nap, so that leaves 12½ hours awake."

CLINICIAN: "So, meals and baths and the like take about an hour and a half a day, and she's gone to school from 8:30 A.M. until 3:30 P.M. That's another 7 hours; she has about 4 hours a day left for everything else in her life?"

MOM: "That sounds about right."

CLINICIAN: "And you say she watches TV at least 2 hours every day? That means that one half of her available time is in front of the tube."

MOM: "Sometimes she plays her video games for a while, too."

CLINICIAN: "Does that seem to you to be leaving enough time for playing and reading and being with the family and everything else you'd like your child to be doing? Does the proportion of her life—50% of her free time—watching TV seem appropriate?"

MOM: "You're making me feel awfully guilty!"

You can write the rest of the dialogue.

Needless to say, there is also the larger, public arena in which we can become involved as advocates for children. We physicians have a long and honorable record of taking active roles in political life, from service on school boards to signing the Declaration of Independence. If Dr. Benjamin Rush could find time to help his country, so can we.

❧ CHAPTER 33

Office-Based Teaching, Research, and Writing

My first thought, when contemplating this chapter, was to start with an eloquent statement proving the importance and utility of office-based academic activity. I was going to argue that the best way to understand a subject was to teach it to someone else. The necessity of a precise and clear grasp of details helps to clarify them in one's own mind. Furthermore, the teacher is forced to keep up to date; one cannot afford to coast forever on the positive information balance last experienced during residency training. For a discussion of research in the setting of practice, I had planned to adduce the advantages of single-observer studies done over many years, a virtual impossibility in medical center–based research. Who else but the practitioner has the chance to do longitudinal studies, observing the same kids over decades of development? Well, as I say, I had planned to make these undoubtedly cogent arguments, but they are somewhat beside the point. The actual reason for the clinical pediatrician to teach and do research is that some of us are driven to do so. Faced with a house officer or a nurse who has a question, we have a palpable need to provide the answer. Contemplating a clinically interesting problem, we begin to fantasize about little research projects to tease out the solutions. This is not necessarily a widely distributed characteristic; some of my best friends in medicine seem immune to the charms of teaching and research. For the nonimmune physician, the opportunities are endless.

Teaching possibilities depend on where you practice and how much time you are willing to contribute; remuneration is unlikely for clinical teachers. If you are near a school of medicine or a teaching hospital, you will have little trouble in finding a place to teach. If your practice has a heavy well-child emphasis, as ours does, inpatient attending teaching is particularly valuable, because it forces you to keep abreast of sick-child pediatrics. We have often had medical students and house officers spending time with us in the office. This allows them to see real-world pediatrics, a universe greatly different from the county hospital or tertiary care hospital in which they have been immersed. We try to show them the relationship and continuing-care aspects of primary pediatric care. Sometimes this includes visits to the newborn in the hospital and a follow-up home call. Having a student with me in the office takes a substantial amount of time. Each visit is prolonged by my asking the student to have a look at that ear or feel that spleen, by the student's interaction with the child and the parent, and by the student's questions after the visit is concluded. If I fail to schedule adequate extra time, I regret it. In our six-doctor office, a visiting student usually spends some time with each of us, which provides a look at the very different ways doctors can manage similar problems. I always ask the parent and child if our visitor may sit in during the consultation, and families are nearly always happy to agree. I have been struck by the obvious pleasure people take in being part of the education of young doctors; they truly enjoy it.

Research projects in practice make sense when the question addressed is rationally connected with the structure of the practice or the particular interests of the doctor. This is nicely exemplified by a study of the inter-relationship of allergic and psychological factors in asthma.[1,2] It was carried out by our founding partner Percy Jennings, a pediatric allergist with a deep interest in family psychology. Our group has long been interested in minimizing the family strains of the newborn period; this led us to do a 14-year study of the feasibility of home phototherapy for hyperbilirubinemia.[3] My unlikely interests in

[1] Jennings PH, et al: Two Components of the Allergic Process Compared: Allergic Potential and Severity of Asthma. J Allergy 1967;39:148–159.
[2] Block J, Jennings P, Harvey E, Simpson E: Interaction Between Allergic Potential and Psychopathology in Childhood Asthma. Psychosom Med 1964;26:307–320.
[3] Rogerson AG, et al: 14 Years of Experience with Home Phototherapy. Clin Pediatr 1986;25:296–302.

teeth and pharmacology came together in a project relating the amount of tetracycline use to the risk and degree of tooth staining.[4] A fondness for relaxation techniques led to a small paper on biofeedback and migraine.[5] An interesting aspect of office-based research is the amazing willingness of parents to participate in these projects. Once we collected babies' stools for a California State Department of Health study of infant botulism. On another occasion we collected blood for a study of influenza vaccination. The tooth-staining study required a visit to the dentist! People really want to help.

Aside from formal research projects, a clinician may develop particular interests and skills that are worth sharing through the medical literature. This is a little tricky, because one's expectation in today's medical environment is that the academicians do the writing and the practitioners do the reading. As a practitioner myself, I always feel somewhat defensive about presuming to submit a paper for publication. When a paper has been rejected by a journal, the comments by the referees who read it are often returned to the author for his enlightenment. On several occasions, I've had the distinct hint that the academicians who looked at my paper found its origin in a private practice rather foreign and offensive. Don't expect every paper you write to find instant acceptance; one of our offerings was rejected three times before it found a home. Despite this impediment, we've had papers published on pediatric practice,[6,7] fluoride,[8] and breastfeeding.[9] For those of us who frequently feel the urge to sound off, book reviews and letters to the editor provide additional and, I believe, useful outlets. Those of us out in the world of medical practice

---

[4]Grossman ER, Walchek A, Freedman H: Tetracyclines and Permanent Teeth: The Relation Between Dose and Tooth Color. Pediatrics 1974;47:567–570.

[5]Peper E, Grossman ER. Thermal Biofeedback Training In Children With Migraine. In Peper E, Ancoli S, Quinn M, eds: Mind-Body Integration: Essential Readings In Biofeedback. New York: Plenum, 1979:489–492.

[6]Jennings P: A Discussion of Certain Opportunities in the Planning of a Pediatric Practice. Pediatrics 1955;15:775–783.

[7]Jennings P: Experience with Prepayment Financing in a Private Pediatric Practice. Pediatr Clin North Am 1969;16:885–889.

[8]Grossman ER: Prescription Use of Fluoride to Control Tooth Decay. G.P. 1963;28:98–102.

[9]Grossman ER: Helping Mothers to Nurse Their Babies. G.P. 1965;31:79–86.

should be an active part of a feedback loop to the world of the medical schools.

Teaching, research, and writing exemplify the wonderful range of opportunities available to us physicians. Within the framework of our everyday pediatric practices, we can study, teach, and try to heal, and we can reach out into our communities. It is hard for me to imagine richer or more satisfying ways to spend a professional life.

Newborn Care and Single-Bottle Formula Making

This is one side of a hand-out given to new mothers; we have it printed on our letterhead.

How to Make Unsterile, Single-Bottle Formula

Your baby's formula need not be sterilized if the milk is safe, the water is obtained from a reliable municipal water supply or other safe sources, and the prepared bottle of formula is used promptly after it is mixed. It *must* be sterilized if water from dubious sources is used or if a whole day's formula is made at one time.

The rules for unsterile formula are as follows:

1. Keep clean, dry bottles in a cupboard, ready to use; nipples and caps can be kept on the bottles or in a covered jar. After a can of liquid formula is opened, cover it with plastic or foil and keep it refrigerated. Dry, powdered formula does not require refrigeration.

2. Make a bottle of formula just before using it; put the formula concentrate in the bottle, add an equal amount of hot tap water, shake it up, and give it to the baby.

3. If the bottle is not used within 2 hours after mixing, throw it away or give it to the cat. Germs (bacteria) will begin to grow in formula after about 2 hours; this will not trouble the cat.

4. If you must take a bottle with you away from home, put powdered formula in the dry bottle, and add the water later when the baby is ready to be fed. Ready-to-use formula in bottles or cans costs more but is even easier.

5. Similac, Enfamil, and other brands of powdered formula are most useful when bottles are used to supplement breast-feeding, to replace breast-feeding on occasion, or when traveling without facilities to refrigerate an open can of milk. Open cans of formula powder last practically forever; ignore the expiration date. Powdered formula is generally mixed as 1 tablespoon of powder for every 2 ounces of warm tap water. Shake vigorously and use. It mixes best if the water is put in the bottle before the powder.

6. The cow's milk–based standard formulas—Similac, Enfamil, SMA, Gerber, and Carnation—are nearly identical. They can be used interchangeably; most babies don't notice the difference.

7. Some formulas come in low-iron as well as iron-fortified forms; the vast majority of infants need the iron-fortified type.

8. Soy formulas differ in digestibility. Isomil, I-Soyalac, Prosobee, and Nursoy are all good products, but some babies do better with one than the others. Soyalac (not I-Soyalac) is somewhat harder for babies to digest. The so-called fresh "soy milks" sold in dairy cold cases are *not* adequate for infant feeding (or anything else).

9. Sugar water is made with 1 teaspoon of white sugar or corn syrup (Karo syrup) per 4 ounces of tap water. Brown sugar may be substituted, but it tends to cause diarrhea. Honey should *not* be used for babies under the age of 1 year; it can cause botulism.

10. If you wish to save breast milk, express it into a clean container and pour the milk into a 4- or 8-ounce nursing bottle. It will keep in the freezer for months. Additional increments of milk can be added to a partly filled bottle.

This is the other side of the formula information form; it is a general new baby information outline with room to write in whatever seems needed by a family.

NURSING

    HOW LONG   HOW OFTEN

    NURSING COMFORT: arm support; arm chair or sofa, pillows
                            baby's position

    NIPPLE CARE: light and air; minimal soap and water

    SUPPLEMENTAL BOTTLE: at least once a week, starting in about
                            2 weeks

FORMULA-FEEDING

SKIN CARE

    BODY: any mild soap; fancy "baby" soaps are not needed

    HEAD AND FACE: any form of baby shampoo

    BATHING FREQUENCY   CARE OF NAVEL

    NO COSMETICS NEEDED; NO POWDER, OIL, CREAM,
      OR LOTIONS

    HOUSE AND ROOM TEMPERATURE

STOOLS

URINE

TAKING CARE OF YOURSELF

    REST

    DIET

    LIMITING VISITORS

    HOUSE CALL   WELL-BABY APPOINTMENTS

Acne Information Sheet

EVERYTHING YOU EVER WANTED TO KNOW ABOUT ACNE AND THEN SOME

What It Is

Acne is a common disorder in which the oil glands of the skin produce an excessive amount of skin oil, and roughening occurs in the lining membranes of the tiny ducts that carry the oil to the surface of the skin. These ducts consequently become partly plugged by dried oil and debris from the duct lining. When a partial obstruction is right at the surface, a blackhead (open comedone) is formed. Where a complete plug forms, a whitehead (closed comedone) develops. The oil trapped within the duct is broken down into irritating fatty acids by the action of skin bacteria. This causes the formation of pimples and small skin abscesses.

These processes tend to develop in adolescence when skin oil production increases in response to changes in sex hormones. The high-sugar diet of the Western world appears to be important in some people, although not in all. Specific skin bacteria play a role as well. As adolescent development is completed in the late teens, the acne process tends to improve spontaneously; in most people, acne disappears by the early twenties.

What Can Be Done

The first thing to understand about acne is that it is a self-limited disorder that will last a few years, and treatment *will not* cure it. The effect of treatment is to suppress the acne until it gradually cures itself. However, a satisfactory degree of control can be obtained by present-day therapy that is properly used. The second rule is that treatment must be tailored to the person, the person's skin, and the kind of acne. For example, a fair-skinned 13-year-old girl needs only very gentle medication; the powerful agents used for severe acne would make her skin worse rather than better. A few years later she might need much more potent medicine if her acne has increased in severity, as often happens.

How to Do It

1. *Hygiene.* Simple face-washing removes skin oils and helps keep oil pores open; warm water, soap, and a washcloth used two times a day can be very helpful, especially in cases of mild acne. Frequent shampooing of the hair helps keep oil off the forehead. Avoiding hair lotions, greases, and oily cosmetics helps, too. Sometimes we suggest using antibacterial soaps like Dial, Safeguard, or pHisoHex. **Scrubs, buffing pads, and abrasives are not helpful and often make acne worse; don't waste your time with them.**

2. *Diet.* Although there has been much debate about the role of food in acne, it is always worth experimenting to see if heavy sugar intake worsens acne. All one has to do is increase candy or soda pop consumption abruptly for a few days. If a large crop of pimples appear, try the reverse experiment of a low-sugar diet for a few weeks. A few people find that a high-fat diet has a deleterious effect.

3. Local treatment, that is, medication applied directly to the skin, encompasses a wide range of liquids, lotions, and gels, which act by scaling off dead skin, opening pores, and exerting a drying effect. **Sulfur, salicylic acid,** and **resorcinol** are the mild agents used for acne of less severity. The mainstay of acne treatment for years has been **benzoyl peroxide,** a drug that works by interfering with the growth of skin bacteria, decreasing the concentration of free fatty acids, and inducing a mild scaling of the skin surface. Bars and washes are the least effective vehicles for benzoyl peroxide; lotions, available without prescription, are quite helpful; gels are much more potent and potentially more irritating; some require a prescription. **Tretinoin (Retin-A)** is a vitamin A–like drug that has the effect of smoothing

the lining of the oil ducts so that old debris can be dislodged, and fewer new plugs form. It must be used cautiously to minimize skin irritation; it also decreases the resistance of the skin to sunburn.

Topical antibiotics are helpful when the skin is irritated and infected around acne-plugged oil glands. **Tetracycline, erythromycin,** and **clindamycin** are all used.

Quite commonly it is best to combine topical medicines; we often suggest benzoyl peroxide or an antibiotic in the morning and tretinoin at bedtime.

4. Systemic treatments are also available. Women with acne can sometimes be helped by certain **birth control pills.** Because of the small but real risk of The Pill, this method is rarely used. **Antibiotics taken by mouth,** usually in small doses, for months to years suppress the growth of bacteria in the oil ducts and usually bring about a substantial decrease in pimples. This use of antibiotics is remarkably safe; side effects are rare and generally easily handled. **Tetracyclines** and **erythromycin** are the usual choices.

The vitamin A–like drug **isotretinoin (Accutane)** is extraordinarily effective against severe acne that has not been controlled by other means. Unlike any other acne treatment, isotretinoin comes close to being a real cure. Unhappily, it has such unpleasant side effects that it must be considered a drug of last resort.

What You Can Expect to Happen

Most people with acne find that they do best when they combine treatments: hygiene, perhaps diet, local medications, and often a systemic antibiotic may eventually all be used. Balancing these agents takes time and attention, from both the patient and the doctor. Many teenagers find it difficult to persist with a years-long undertaking like this, in which improvement is slow and many changes of treatment may be needed. It is easy to give up, forget to use the medicine, or try some magical and highly advertised cure recommended by a friend. However, the reward for perseverance is the clearest-possible skin during adolescence and the least-possible acne scarring to carry into adult life.

❦ APPENDIX C

Safety Grid for Floor Heaters

Attach dowels to upright boards with small nails or screws or, preferably, holes in boards and glue dowels in place.

Safety grid can be anchored to the floor with steel angle-irons and screws or simply wired down to the heater top.

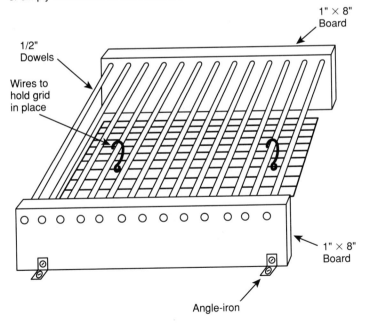

1" × 8"
Board

1/2"
Dowels

Wires to
hold grid
in place

1" × 8"
Board

Angle-iron

❧ INDEX